MW00814675

I Have IBS...
Now What?!!!

A Comprehensive Guide for Patients with
Irritable Bowel Syndrome

Dr. Ashkan Farhadi, MD, MS
Senior Member of the
American College of Gastroenterology

SanitizAir Inc.
Version E4
2008

Dedicated To:
My wonderful wife Ziba who is the wind beneath my wings.
My Children, Argi and Nili Who are the joy of my life and
My parents, without you I would not be ...

CONTENTS

FOREWORD

The goal of this book is to increase your basic knowledge about Irritable Bowel Syndrome (IBS) and potential treatments of this common problem. In this book, I have tried to elaborate on several aspects of this disorder and to answer frequently asked questions. The format of the book is "question and answer" or "Q and A". These are real questions and answers that have been asked by my patients and answered by me. The format is very similar to what occurs during a typical visit to your physician's office. Thus, you could save a lot of time and money by going through this book. Additionally, in an effort to enable individuals with a non-medical background to understand the basic concepts of IBS, the language of the book is straightforward.

There are currently numerous publications that address Irritable Bowel Syndrome. Many of them are good resources for patients with IBS and most of them are quite comprehensive. The advantage of my book over other publications is in the simplicity of the content and emphasis on subtle but important issues that you confront in your daily life. I tried to avoid discussing complicated and impractical issues to ensure that you will easily grasp the major issues related to IBS. My aim is to create in your mind a realistic impression of the disorder. This knowledge will not only improve your understanding of the disorder, but also, it will provide you with new insights into treatment options. I believe this simple but broad view of the disorder will reduce most of your fears and anxiety about IBS and offer you increased confidence and control over your illness.

The idea and inspiration for this book occurred to me

while I was answering questions that IBS patients usually raise during typical office visits. I thought that by putting these questions and answers in a small booklet, I would save a lot of time for both my patients and myself. I never intended to publish this book on a large-scale basis. However, within a short time, 10,000 copies of the first edition were sold and the second edition was published shortly thereafter. The book was very successful and received extremely positive feedback. In this edition, I present the most up to date information and recent advances in the field. I also used the help of several consultants in writing this new edition. Adding their knowledge as well as more than 10 years of my experience in diagnosis, treatment and research in this field, I believe this book presents cutting-edge information about IBS in simple terms and will help you to understand the problem. This knowledge will not only increase your coping capability, it will help you to be an effective part of a management team. Although I use a lot of medical terminology and jargon that you may have already heard of in your numerous medical encounters, simple explanations of these terms are presented throughout the book.

The creation of this book has been a wonderful project and was accomplished because of the contributions of many individuals. In particular are all of the patients who shared their stories with me, who were a real inspiration for this project. Also, I am very grateful to my consultants who shared their wisdom and knowledge.

Dr. Ashkan Farhadi, MD
Master of Sciences in Clinical Research
Senior Member of the American College of Gastroenterology

INTRODUCTION (GENERAL FACTS)

Irritable bowel syndrome (IBS) is defined as a functional bowel disorder in which abdominal pain is associated with changes in bowel habits.[1, 2] Peters first coined the term Irritable Bowel Syndrome in 1944, and since then, our knowledge of the syndrome has increased significantly.[3] However, physicians and patients have been using many different terms to describe this common problem for years. These names include mucus colitis, spastic colon, nervous colitis, nervous bowel disease, irritable colon and functional bowel disorder. I will use only IBS.

Research indicates that IBS is the most common disorder of the gastrointestinal tract. The overall prevalence of IBS in the general population in the United States is approximately 10% (1 in 10 people have IBS), although individual studies report prevalence rates that vary widely, ranging from 3% to 22%.[4-9] The reason for this variation is due in part to the diversity of the IBS definitions used and the methods of information gathering.

IBS accounts for one third of gastroenterology office visits and is a frequent reason for office visits to primary care physicians.[4] IBS is a disorder that causes emotional distress, lower quality of life, and increased health-care costs. Despite our growing knowledge about the syndrome, IBS remains a disorder that is not fully understood. Moreover, a wide range of symptoms of this disorder is similar to symptoms of other gastrointestinal disorders. This can lead to a great deal of confusion among patients and physicians and eventually results in frustration and disappointment. Unfortunately, following unsuccessful treatments, most of these patients are disheartened and find themselves wandering from one medical office to another, in search of a crystal-clear diagnosis and treatment.

Here, I will try to provide a thorough review of this disorder while keeping the language simple. To this end, I will present a clear perspective on the mechanisms that cause the disorder, on the symptoms, and on the methods used to diagnose IBS. I will also discuss a variety of conventional and alternative therapies that already exist for this disorder, while referring to newer therapies that may become more common in the future.

Consultants

- ## Michael D. Brown, MD, FACP, FACG
  Dr. Michael Brown is an Associate Professor of Medicine, Gastroenterologist and the Director of the Fellowship Program in the Section of Gastroenterology & Nutrition at Rush University Medical Center in Chicago, IL.

- ## Sharon Jedel, PsyD
  Dr. Sharon Jedel is a Clinical Psychologist in the Section of Gastroenterology & Nutrition at Rush University Medical Center in Chicago, IL.

- ## Mary C. Tobin, MD
  Dr. Tobin is an Assistant Professor of Medicine, and specialist in allergy and immunology at Rush University Medical Center in Chicago, IL.

- ## Andrea Borowiecki, MPH, CHES
  Andrea Borowiecki is the Program Marketing Manager for the Section of Gastroenterology & Nutrition at Rush University Medical Center in Chicago.

- ## Douglas A. Drossman, MD
  Dr. Douglas Drossman is a Professor of Medicine and Psychiatry, Co-director, University of North Carolina Center for Functional GI and Motility Disorders in Chapel Hill, NC.

- ## Susan L. Mikolaitis, RD, LDN, CSND
  Susan L. Mikolaitis is a registered dietitian with more than 20 years of experience in nutrition therapy for gastrointestinal diseases at Rush University Medical Center in Chicago.

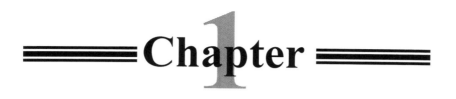

Chapter 1

DEFINITION
(NAMING THE DISORDER, RIGHT OR WRONG)

In this chapter, you will learn:

✓   _What "Irritable Bowel Syndrome" is._

✓   _What "Functional Bowel Disorder" is._

✓   _What "normal looking" bowel means._

✓   _An exact definition of IBS._

✓   _Why IBS is considered a "syndrome" and not a disease._

❖ **What is "Irritable Bowel Syndrome"?**

Irritable Bowel Syndrome or IBS is a type of functional bowel disorder that is characterized by abdominal pain and change in bowel habits.

❖ **What is a "Functional Bowel Disorder"?**

Gastrointestinal or GI tract disorders include two major categories: organic GI disorders and functional bowel disorders. Subjects with organic GI disorders have either gross abnormalities, like a tumor, ulcer or inflammation, or microscopic abnormalities. Subjects with "functional" bowel disorders, on the contrary, do not have any visible or microscopic problem in their GI tracts. In fact, functional bowel disorders all have a "normal looking gastrointestinal tract".

❖ **What does "normal looking" mean?**

It means that if one were to look at the GI tract with the naked eye (during an endoscopic procedure), it would appear normal. An endoscope is a fiberoptic instrument that enables doctors to have a close look at the GI mucosa (the lining of your bowel). This instrument also makes it possible for the physician to obtain tissue samples from the gastrointestinal mucosa, a procedure called mucosal biopsy, which serves for microscopic examination of the intestine. In IBS, despite a normal looking appearance of the GI tract, the bowel does not function normally. In functional bowel disease, the main problem is related to disturbed motility and sensitivity.

❖ **Does this mean that a person with a GI problem has**

either an <u>**organic**</u> GI disorder or a <u>**functional**</u> bowel disorder?

Not exactly. There can be some overlap. For example, there are many people who suffer from both Inflammatory Bowel Disease (i.e., Crohn's disease or Ulcerative Colitis) and IBS. In this situation, it is not uncommon to see symptoms, which continue even when the inflammation is well under control. For example, let's say that Mark has Inflammatory Bowel Disease and after successful medical management and

Figure 1: Classification of GI disorders

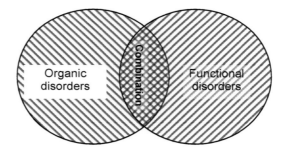

when the inflammation in his bowel is well under control, his symptoms, such as diarrhea and cramps persist. These symptoms may now represent a component of IBS "see Figure 1."

❖   **So, IBS is one of the functional bowel disorders. What are other functional bowel disorders?**

There is a bunch of them. Common functional disorders include non-ulcer dyspepsia, painless constipation, painless diarrhea, irritable esophagus and chronic abdominal pain "see Figure 2."

Figure 2: Classification of functional GI

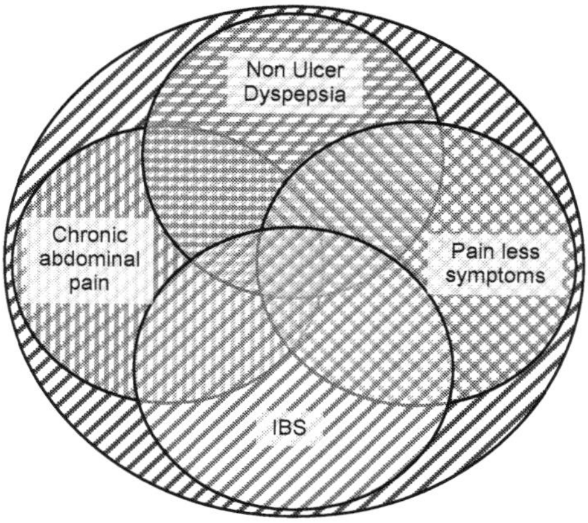

❖   **What is the exact definition of IBS?**

One of the first definitions of IBS was proposed in 1978 by Dr. Manning and his colleagues who recommended that a diagnosis of IBS be based on the presence of the following four symptoms; 1) pain that is improved after a bowel movement, 2) diarrhea at the onset of abdominal pain, 3) more frequent bowel movements at the onset of pain and 4) visible abdominal distension (bloating).[10] These symptoms differentiate patients with IBS from patients with organic diseases. About ten years later, a group of physicians gathered in Rome and proposed new criteria for the diagnosis of IBS (the Rome-I criteria). The Rome-I criteria (1992) and subsequently the Rome-II (1999) and Rome-III (2006) criteria have added to our understanding of IBS. According to these criteria, IBS is defined as recurrent abdominal pain or discomfort at least 3 days/month in last 3 months associated with two or more of the following features: 1) relief upon having a bowel movement, 2) onset associated with a change in frequency of bowel movement or 3) onset associated with change in the form or appearance of the stool. The symptoms must be present for at least 3 Months (which do not need to be consecutive) over the past 6 months.[11, 12] Only a few physicians currently rely on the Rome criteria for diagnostic purposes. However, these criteria are well established among researchers who do clinical studies on IBS.

❖ **What are the other names for IBS?**

There are several other names for this disorder that you may have heard before. These include nervous colitis, spastic colon, mucus colitis, irritable colon and nervous bowel disease. However, none of these terms is appropriate for this disorder.

❖ **Why is the terminology "Irritable Bowel Syndrome" preferable to other terms, such as "colitis"?**

Colitis means inflammation of the colon (large bowel). There is no endoscopic inflammation in IBS. Therefore, it is not appropriate to use the term colitis for IBS.

❖ **So, why is IBS considered a "syndrome" and not a disease?**

A syndrome is a collection of signs and symptoms that cannot be explained by a specific underlying mechanism. For example, in IBS, we do not know why people may have both gastrointestinal and non-gastrointestinal symptoms at the same time. In fact, certain diseases, such as peptic ulcers or infectious disease, can present with some of the same symptoms. Typically, we do not know exactly why or how this collection occurs. This is why we call it "syndrome."

❖ **Is IBS more common among men or women?**

IBS is more prevalent among women. For example, a study in the United Kingdom indicated a prevalence of 13% in women and 5% in men.[9]

❖ **I had my symptoms for 4 weeks last year and this year similar symptoms lasted for 6 weeks. However, according to the definition you mentioned earlier, I do not have IBS. So what do I have?**

According to the Rome-III criteria, you have a functional bowel disorder. However, I believe that the main reason for proposing such criteria was for better differentiating patients who suffer from short-term or acute gastrointestinal infectious disorders from patients who suffer from a chronic process, such as IBS. This classification also might be very useful for scientists for research purposes (such as drug studies), or physicians and office administrators for billing purposes. I do not see any clear-cut difference between someone whose symptoms have occurred for 10 weeks versus someone with symptoms for 12 weeks.

❖ **I have abdominal pain that is relieved by defecation. However, my stools are not really loose. So, it seems I meet one of the Manning criteria or the Rome-III criteria. Do I have IBS?**

Dr. Farhadi: According to this definition, no. However, I do not consider the Manning and Rome criteria to be written in stone. Whether these symptoms are labeled IBS or not, the underlying process is the same.

Dr. Drossman: Possibly. It is not uncommon for

individuals to experience pain and bowel symptoms like diarrhea in response to stress, diary indiscretion, hormonal changes like having a menstrual period, physical exercise and the like. IBS can be understood as a disorder where there is an increased sensitivity to react to such factors. It also occurs frequently and for a period of time. If you have had these symptoms in the past, it is more likely you have IBS. The Rome III criteria for diagnosing IBS includes [13, 14]: • Recurrent abdominal pain or discomfort at least 3 days/month in last 3 months associated with two or more: • Improvement with defecation; • Onset associated with a change in frequency of stool; • Onset associated with a change in form (appearance) of stool. These criteria need to be fulfilled for the last 3 months with symptom onset at least 6 months prior to diagnosis.

❖ **I have bloating and a severe urge to have a bowel movement after eating. This is not one of the criteria for IBS. Do I still have IBS?**

My answer is the same as for the previous question. Indeed, as you will see throughout the book, whenever I use the term IBS, I am considering a broader definition, which is more far-reaching than the Manning, Rome-I, Rome-II and Rome III criteria. By using this term, I am referring to a **sensitive bowel**, which responds abnormally to **irritant stimuli.** I do not believe there is a clear distinction between the different functional bowel disorders "see Figure 2." In fact, many patients have symptoms of different functional bowel disorders at the same time and we are therefore unable to diagnose them as having one specific syndrome.

❖ **Based on this broader definition, how many people have IBS?**

This is difficult to answer and I am not entirely sure. I think that many people out there suffer from one or more IBS symptoms but these symptoms are not troubling them enough to seek further medical attention. If we used the broader definition of IBS, imagine how many more people would fit into this new definition!

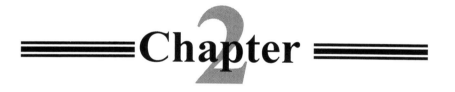

Chapter 2

ETIOLOGY
(NATURE OF THE DISORDER)

In this chapter, you will learn:

✓   *What causes Irritable Bowel Syndrome.*

✓   *What the irritant stimuli are.*

✓   *How the irritant stimuli cause symptoms.*

✓   *Why your abdominal pain changes places.*

✓   *Whether this disorder only affects your bowel.*

✓   *What the role of mast cells is in IBS.*

✓   *Whether food allergy is related to IBS.*

❖   **What causes Irritable Bowel Syndrome?**

IBS is the result of a **sensitive bowel**, which responds abnormally to **irritant stimuli**. In fact, IBS symptoms origin from a blend of **abnormal intestinal motility** or movement and **abnormal intestinal sensation**.

❖   **What are the irritant stimuli that cause IBS?**

There are several irritant stimuli "see Figure 3."

Figure 3: Common stimuli that trigger IBS symptoms

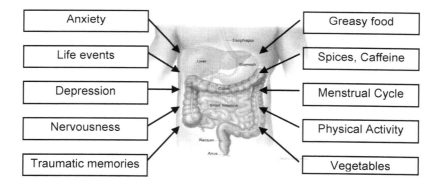

Anxiety	Greasy food
Life events	Spices, Caffeine
Depression	Menstrual Cycle
Nervousness	Physical Activity
Traumatic memories	Vegetables

❖   **If these are not all of the irritant stimuli what else is there?**

That is a tricky question. This diagram only gives you a general idea of what the irritant stimuli could be. However, in reality, the triggers could be a mixture of these and other stimuli. You may be in the best position to detect your specific stimuli.

❖   **Are all of the patients affected by all of these stimuli?**

No. Each individual is usually affected by just one or two

of these irritant stimuli. Only a small fraction of patients is affected by more than a few stimuli. Furthermore, the symptoms are usually triggered by a mixture of these stimuli such as psychological and food stimuli. In this case, there is usually one major irritant stimulus.

❖   **Do all people respond in the same way to these stimuli?**

Absolutely not. One IBS patient may experience abdominal pain in response to specific food while another IBS patient may experience diarrhea.

❖   **How do these stimuli cause symptoms?**

To answer this question, I first have to explain briefly the function of the gastrointestinal or GI tract. The GI tract moves food from the stomach into the small bowel (small intestine) and eventually into the large bowel (colon). This movement is called peristalsis and is regulated at two levels. The first level is in the intestine and is called the enteric nervous system. The second level is in the brain, which is part of the central nervous system. These two regulatory systems are closely linked. This whole system is called the Brain Gut Axis (BGA). This axis transfers information from the brain to The GI tract and from the GI tract back to the brain. The first is called the efferent pathway; the second the afferent pathway.

Now let me get back to your question. The basic answer is that stimuli can trigger the pain by affecting the brain gut axis.

❖   **What does the Brain-Gut-Axis do?**

Figure 4: A schematic representation of the Brain Gut Axis

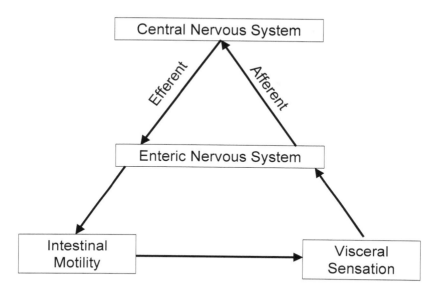

As you can see in Figure 4, the central nervous system is connected to what is called the enteric nervous system (another name for the collection of nerve cells in the GI tract) through the Vagus nerve and sympathetic nerves "see Figure 4." This connection allows exchange of information between the central and enteric nervous systems. There are receptors in the gut that can sense pain and pressure. When the bowel is irritated, these receptors convey this information to the brain through the afferent pathway of the BGA. The brain also can control the functions of the GI tract, such as digestion, secretion, absorption and movement of the bowel through the efferent pathways of the BGA. Food stimuli usually affect the afferent pathways while psychological stimuli usually affect efferent pathways.

❖   **How does the exchange of data between the afferent and efferent pathways take place in the BGA?**

The exchange of data between the central and the enteric nervous systems occurs through the afferent and efferent pathways. The nerves convey the data in a similar way that information is transferred through the electrical wires in your computer. The data travels along nerves as electrical impulses. The data is transferred from one nerve to another as chemical impulses. The latter occurs in the spaces between nerve terminals called synapses. When an electrical impulse reaches the end of the nerve (also known as a pre-synaptic nerve ending), a chemical agent is released from the nerve ending into the synaptic space. The chemical agent is called a neurotransmitter. Thousands to millions of the neurotransmitter molecules travel through the synaptic space to the nerve on the other side (also known as the post-synaptic nerve) and attaches to large protein molecules called receptors. The receptor is like a lock and the neurotransmitter is like a key that opens the lock. Activation of the post-synaptic receptors triggers an electrical impulse in the postsynaptic nerve. This is how an electrical

Figure 5: How electrical nerve impulses pass to the other nerves through release of chemical neurotransmitters at the terminal end of nerves (synapses)

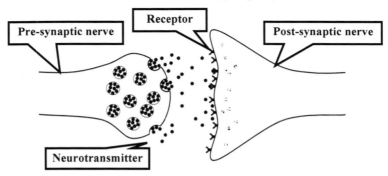

impulse "jumps" from one nerve to another "see Figure 5."

Serotonin is one of these neurotransmitters. In fact, it is the most important neurotransmitter in the BGA. Now comes the interesting part! The same neurotransmitter can actually convey different messages to the post-synaptic nerve. How? The type of receptor in the post-synaptic nerve determines the type of response that occurs from the neurotransmitter. This property of the neurotransmitter and different type of receptors are the basis for discoveries of new drugs. For example, a medicine that blocks type 3 serotonin receptor can result in a decrease of gastrointestinal movement (constipation) while a medicine that stimulates the type 4 serotonin receptor can cause increasing gastrointestinal movement (diarrhea). (Isn't that weird?).

❖ **This is getting too complicated. Serotonin, synapse, and now varieties of receptors. What is the use of all this information?**

This basic knowledge will help you to better understand the mechanisms of Irritable Bowel Syndrome. When you are considering therapeutic options, it is important to have an overview of these mechanisms. Most of the new medications that are prescribed these days work through these receptor pathways.

❖ **How does the abnormal movement of the bowel create so many varieties of symptoms in IBS?**

Good question! It helps to have an example. A prolonged severe simultaneous contraction (spasm) in some part of the GI tract particularly at the end of the large bowel can produce pain and constipation. On the other hand, a forceful peristalsis or forward movement of the bowel can result in a rapid emptying of the bowel content, causing diarrhea.

❖ **Why does my abdominal pain change places?**

The GI tract is one of the major organs inside the abdomen that fills most of the space inside the abdominal cavity. A spasm in different parts of the GI tract can produce pain in different areas of the abdomen. For example, a spasm of the gastro-duodenal portion (the stomach and the first part of the small intestine) may be experienced in the epigastric area (the middle of the upper abdomen, just below the chest bone). A small intestinal spasm may be experienced around the umbilicus (the belly button) and a spasm in the colon may be experienced in either side of the lower abdomen, depending on the presence of a spasm in the right or left side of the colon. Furthermore, pain is not restricted to these areas and may be experienced in other parts of the abdomen as well as simultaneously in several different places.

❖ **Is a spasm always associated with pain?**

No. As mentioned above, motility problems result in a wide variety of symptoms, not just pain. For example, many individuals complain of bloating, fullness, diarrhea and/or constipation.

❖ **I have no problem with intestinal motility. My main issue is pain. Is it possible to have pain without motility difficulties?**

IBS is a mixture of dysmotility (abnormal intestinal movement) and hypersensitivity (abnormal intestinal sensation).

In another word, IBS is based on an intestinal "dysmotility-hypersensitivity" model. These two key features are at the opposite ends of the IBS spectrum. We can locate most of the problems of IBS somewhere in the middle of this spectrum "see Figure 6."

Figure 6: Spectrum of symptoms in relation to abnormalities in IBS

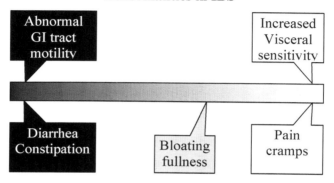

At one end of the spectrum are individuals who have normal intestinal motility with extreme hypersensitivity. These individuals may feel pain with minimal or even normal intestinal contractions. On the other end of the spectrum are individuals who have abnormal intestinal motility without hypersensitivity. These individuals may experience many intestinal contractions without any abdominal pain or discomfort, and usually have painless diarrhea or constipation. In the middle are individuals who experience a little of both abnormalities and thus, experience both group of symptoms.

❖   **If one or a few stimuli are triggering my symptoms, how come my symptoms do not always occur with the same stimuli? In other words, why do I have symptoms "off and on"?**

As you may recall, symptoms are due to environmental stimuli. Most often, the presence of one stimulus alone is not strong enough to trigger symptoms; however, a combination of two or more stimuli can trigger symptoms. For example, consider Mary, a college student majoring in literature. During final exams, she experiences abdominal pain, bloating and diarrhea only when consuming spicy foods. She never had difficulties with spicy food in the past. In Mary's case, it is a combination of two stimuli such as spicy food and exam stress, which cause her symptoms. This is why, combined stimuli create a major problem in identifying the primary stimulus that triggers IBS symptoms.

❖   **I recently attended my sister's wedding, which was one of the happiest days of my life. I do not have any psychological problems but I experienced severe abdominal pain that day. Why did this happen?**

Psychological stimuli are not limited to depression and sadness. Any changes in one's lifestyle or environment, whether good or bad, could result in anxiety and stress, which are very potent stimuli.

❖   **So, you are telling me that despite all pain, bloating and other symptoms, I have a normal GI tract!?**

Yes and no! Your GI tract would have looked normal if you had been examined with a series of conventional diagnostic tests, including endoscopy, colonoscopy, X-rays and lab tests.

❖   **So, I am healthy?**

Sort of. Your GI tract looks normal. However, despite a normal appearance, this system has functional problems, which results in IBS symptoms.

❖ **I have been referred to several physicians and after extensive evaluation, they told me "you are healthy and everything is in your head". But, I am sure that there is something wrong with me. So, I kept changing doctors to figure out my problem. Are you telling me now that I have a real problem in my GI tract?**

Yes. Actually, acceptance and understanding of your disorder is one of the key steps in your successful treatment.

❖ **Finally, after all these years, I feel a little bit better now that I know that I have a common, treatable disorder. Everybody thought that everything was in my head and that I think I am sick, or "psycho" or that I like to play the sick role. So, they were wrong!**

Yes. IBS is very well known to most physicians. It is even possible to observe the abnormalities in GI motility when certain sophisticated types of tests are conducted. However, due to various complexities associated with administering these tests, they are not routinely performed. Thus, the diagnosis of IBS is primarily based on clinical data, including a detailed history, thorough physical exam, and simple lab tests.

❖ **I have had this disorder for many years and I think it is the disorder that is making me nervous, rather than my nervousness causing the disorder. What do you think?**

You might be right "see Figure 7."

Figure 7: The IBS vicious cycle

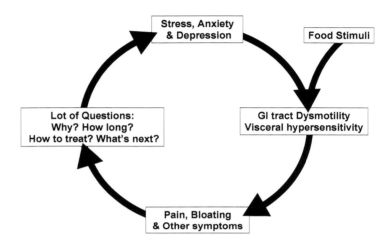

As I mentioned earlier, IBS is the result of GI tract dysmotility and hypersensitivity. Psychological, food and environmental stimuli can result in pain, bloating, fullness and other symptoms. Consequently, one asks questions such as, what is going on? What is causing these problems? Is it a serious problem? Do I have cancer? How long will it last? Will it resolve on its own or is there a quick fix to it? Such questions and related concerns can themselves result in stress and anxiety. As you see, the vicious cycle is now complete! Now, the question is which comes first, the chicken or the egg?

❖   **So, you are telling me that all of my problems come from environmental stimuli. But, why only me? There are many other people in my exact situation who do not have these problems.**

We really don't know what causes people who live in

similar environmental conditions to have different health problems. Certainly, genetic factors play an important role. For example, your central or enteric nervous system may be significantly more sensitive to stimuli compared to others. For sure, your body's structure and response to environmental stimuli is not similar to other people. However, we cannot blame everything on genetics. We believe that various environmental factors, such as infections, stress and food can result in changes in the BGA and intestinal tract causing hypersensitivity or dysmotility. The bottom line is that in order for IBS to develop, you need a GI tract that is more sensitive to irritant stimuli and the presence of triggering stimuli. Individually, neither of these two factors alone is capable of creating IBS symptoms.

❖ **Does this disorder affect only my bowel?**

No. As I mentioned earlier, this disorder can have extra-intestinal symptoms involving organs outside the GI tract. It seems that most organs that are regulated by the autonomic nervous system can have similar functional problems. For example, abnormal contraction of the smooth muscle in the wall of the urinary bladder can manifest itself as urinary frequency; similarly, abnormal smooth muscle contraction in the uterus can result in painful menstruation (dysmenorrhea). Thus, you may experience a variety of extra-intestinal symptoms.

❖ **I wonder whether all symptoms are equally related to the same stimuli.**

No. For example, abdominal pain, diarrhea and bloating may be related to food intake, while constipation, flatulence, and incomplete evacuation (a sense of incomplete bowel movements) are usually not related to food intake.

❖   **My doctor told me that my symptoms might be related to some infection in my stomach. What do you think?**

Several studies have indicated an association between Non-Ulcer Dyspepsia and the presence of a bacterium in the stomach, which is called Helicobacter Pylori. Non-Ulcer Dyspepsia is another functional bowel disease that mainly presents with pain in the upper part of the abdomen and dyspepsia. I should mention that this infection is the most common infection in the world, and up to 20% of healthy individuals in the United States have this infection in their stomach. In other countries, this infection is even more prevalent and rates are as high as 70-80%. So far, studies have not indicated that eradication of this bacterium results in a long-term improvement of symptoms in Non-Ulcer Dyspepsia. Nevertheless, this bacterium should be eradicated. This is because not only it can cause peptic ulceration, but it also can result in gastric cancer. There is some connection between IBS and Non-Ulcer Dyspepsia. In fact, in one study, those subjects with IBS who had dyspeptic symptoms had a higher rate of H. Pylori infection.[15] But in general, there is no clear relationship between H. Pylori and IBS.

❖   **I was completely healthy until my trip to New Mexico last year, where I had an awful case of gastroenteritis for a few days. Since then, I have been suffering from IBS. Nothing in my environment, including food or stress, has changed over the last year. So why do I have IBS now and not before my trip?**

Tough question! A limited number of studies report the occurrence of IBS following infectious gastroenteritis (post-infectious IBS). Let's get back to the "hypersensitivity - dysmotility" model. Infections usually result in accumulation of inflammatory cells, which release their mediators or cytokines. These compounds can affect the local nerves and increase their sensitivity. For example, suppose you were burned on your arm. The area surrounding the burn is usually supersensitive to touch and painful stimuli. This is due to the effect of inflammatory cells, and the chemicals they release (cytokines). These cytokines can affect the enteric nervous system in the GI tract and result in disturbances in the system's functioning. This causes abdominal pain and diarrhea during acute gastroenteritis. In most cases, inflammation-induced changes are part of a transient process that diminishes once the infection is resolved and inflammation subsides. In some cases, the effect of this inflammatory process persists in the form of disturbed sensitivity and motility of the bowel, despite the fact that most of the inflammation has been resolved. In such cases, the stimuli that did not cause pain and dysmotility before, are now capable of doing so and causing symptoms.

Bear in mind that post-infectious IBS only comprises a small minority of IBS cases and that the overwhelming majority of patients with IBS do not fit into this category.

❖ **So, is the increased sensitivity of my bowel only due to irritation of the afferent pathway of the BGA?**

No. The increased sensitivity of the bowel can occur due to various problems associated with the BGA.

In the example above, that individual experienced irritation of nerve endings in the afferent pathway of the BGA due to cytokines. Release of other chemicals such as serotonin and mast cells mediators can result in intestinal hypersensitivity. On the

Figure 8: The relationship of pain sensation and severity of stimuli.

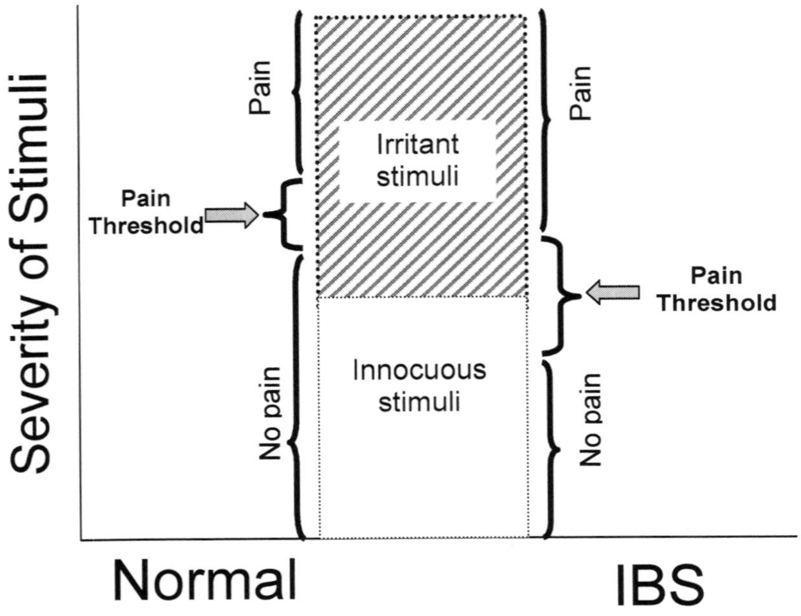

other hand, many IBS patients have problems with central components of the BGA or the brain.

A glance at Figure 8 shows that in normal people, not all of the irritant stimuli could result in pain sensation. Why? There is a pain inhibitory center within the brain that can suppress the sensation of pain. This area uses chemicals such as locally made narcotics (Endorphins) and other neurotransmitters to "trick" your mind into thinking that you are not experiencing the pain. In normal people, non-painful (innocuous) stimuli do not result in pain. However, among patients with IBS, the pain center malfunction may result in increased pain sensation with minimal irritant stimuli, which is called hyperalgesia. In severe cases of IBS, even innocuous stimuli can result in pain (allodynia). Thus, even normal motility following a normal meal can result in pain. Emotions, feelings, and stress can modify the function of this inhibitory center and it is not surprising that psychological well-being has an important impact on the magnitude and severity of the perceived pain.

❖ **I have heard that a ton of bacteria live in the intestinal tract. Is that true? And if so, what is the role of intestinal bacteria in IBS?**

The intestinal tract is the largest surface that connects the human body with the external environment. More than 2000 square feet of the intestinal surface is exposed to food, and thus it is not unusual that various groups of bacteria live in different parts of the GI tract. For example, the number of bacteria in the mouth is close to 100 billion colonies per cubic millimeter of saliva. There is a similar amount of bacteria in the large bowel and stool. These bacteria are normal flora (good bacteria) and have a mutually helpful (symbiotic) relationship with the body. In fact, they protect our bodies from invasion of bad bacteria. Due to the acidic environment of the stomach as well as the digestive enzymes in the small bowel, the environment of the stomach and the small bowel is almost germ-free. Recently, researchers have proposed that one of the culprits that cause IBS is an imbalance of good and bad bacteria in the large intestine.[16] This imbalance does not take the form of gastroenteritis or acute diarrheal illness, but results in abnormalities in the level of cytokines. In one study, this imbalance of cytokines was reversed when the good bacteria in the bowel were restored.[16]

❖ **Last summer I went bankrupt. I was under a huge amount of stress for a while when my IBS symptoms started. Now, I am back at work and doing well financially. I no longer have the stress from before but I still have the same symptoms. How do you explain my situation with your stimuli-symptom theory?**

Before answering this question, let me discuss some new research on the role of stress in GI tract disorders. I should mention that this area of research is one of the least explored areas of GI physiology. Some investigators have studied the relationship between stress and the GI tract among rats (rats hate water and their fear of drowning produces significant stress). These studies have found that after 5 days of exposure to the stressful situation of forced swimming, the number of mast cells in the rats' intestine increased.[17, 18]

Now, you may ask, what is a mast cell? Mast cells are some of the intermediaries in the chain of command of the brain-gut axis. In fact, these cells represent one of the most important end effectors of the BGA in the GI tract and release numerous chemical mediators and cytokines in response to increased activity of efferent BGA nerves (BGA output). These mediators change the sensitivity of sensory nerves, intestinal barrier integrity, intestinal immune properties, intestinal motility and many other intestinal functions.[19] Among a wide range of physiological effects of chemicals released from mast cells into the GI tract is an increased sensitivity of sensory terminals of the afferent BGA (BGA input). The increased activity of the afferent sensory nerves could result in increased BGA activity, which in turn results in increased output of this system in the form of increased discharge of the efferent nerves of the BGA. The increased discharge of the efferent nerves of the BGA translates into an increase in the release of mast cell mediators. Guess what? This creates another self-amplifying loop or vicious cycle in the IBS. So let me now rephrase your question: "If I am exposed to stress, is the effect of stress on my body transient or permanent?" There is no clear answer to this question at the present time. See Figure 7 to understand how stress affects the gastrointestinal tract and creates a vicious cycle that can persist even in the absence of initiating factors.

❖ **What about mast cells in the human GI tract? What is their role in IBS?**

There are only a few studies on human subjects that address this issue. My colleagues and I recently published a study on the role of stress among healthy volunteers.[20] We found that the number of mast cells in the mucosa of the colon only increased minimally after subjects were exposed to a stressful situation – putting their hand in ice-cold water for 15 minutes each day for 5 consecutive days. This procedure causes severe pain and served as the source of stress in our study (cruel, isn't it?). We investigated the effects of this stressful situation on the gastrointestinal tracts of the subjects. Our results indicated that when people experience stressful situations, mast cells at the end of the BGA axis (in the GI tract) release their mediators into the gastrointestinal mucosa, and this is associated with mucosal cell damage. So, is it possible to apply these findings to IBS?

Not exactly. However, they do suggest that structural changes occur in the GI tract after repeated stress. Other studies have found that subjects with IBS have more mast cells in the small bowel mucosa and that these cells are in close proximity to the sensory afferent nerves of the mucosa.[21, 22] There are also a few reports of IBS patients with severe symptoms who had an abundance of mast cells in the mucosa of their small bowel. This condition is known as mast cell enterocolitis.[23]

❖   **So, are you saying that stress can cause permanent changes and damage to my intestine?**

At this point, our scientific knowledge on the effect of stress on the GI tract is limited and we cannot state with certainty how long the effect of stress on the GI tract persists in each individual. In most individuals, the effect of stress on the body is transient and will eventually diminish. However, the effect of stress can persist in the form of unpleasant memories or reoccurring thoughts. For example, having memories of being abused as a child can stay with you and cause long-term effects.

❖   **I have some bad memories from my childhood. Do you think my current problem with IBS has to do any thing with those thoughts?**

Dr. Drossman: IBS is a disorder where the symptoms of pain, diarrhea and constipation can be influenced by thoughts and feelings.[24, 25] This is no surprise; it is common to get bowel symptoms when under stress, like before giving a presentation, traveling, or when experiencing something that is emotionally disturbing, like sexual or physical abuse, or losing a loved one. Conversely, the mind has the ability to suppress pain and other symptoms through hypnosis, focused meditation or relaxation. We call this the "brain-gut" connection. There is now scientific evidence to show that early bad memories from childhood including abuse, emotional deprivation, abandonment or major losses can contribute to gastrointestinal or other symptoms later in life.[26, 27] Rather than actually causing IBS, we believe that traumatic experiences and the emotions trigger physiological changes in the brain that impair its ability to regulate these symptoms. In these cases, antidepressants and psychological treatments may be helpful.

❖ **Is stress the only psychological stimulus that affects my symptoms?**

Unfortunately, no. Stress and anxiety can happen during major disruptive life events such as divorce, death of a loved one, or loss of job. Stress and anxiety can also happen throughout minor life events and even during daily activities such as hassles at home or in the work place. In fact, as I mentioned above, any changes in one's lifestyle or environment, whether good or bad, can result in anxiety and stress. Stress and anxiety may result from unpleasant memories or reoccurring thoughts; this is particularly true regarding earlier life experiences, like childhood abuse. In addition to stress and anxiety induced by major and minor life events, other psychological stimuli or conditions can play a role in the development and course of IBS. These include depression, chronic pain, perimenstrual (around menstrual period) tension and insomnia. You also should bear in mind that depending on the strength of individual coping mechanisms, the effect of environmental stress on the body varies greatly. We will discuss this in details in the chapter on IBS treatments.

❖ **I saw my allergy doctor and he was explaining my allergic disease and used the term "mast cells" very often. Is this the same type of mast cell you are talking about?**

Yes. In fact, mast cells have several different functions in the body. They play a vital role in the initiation and persistence of allergies, protecting the body against infectious agents and activating the body's immune system.[19]

❖ **Are allergic rhinitis (stuffy and runny nose due to allergy) and other types of allergies related to IBS?**

My colleagues and I recently conducted a research study and found that allergic disorders are closely associated with IBS. Data from this study indicated that subjects with IBS have a higher incidence of allergies.[28] Similarly, subjects with allergic disorders have a higher incidence of IBS. This finding is not surprising since both disorders share mast cells as one of their key elements. As a result of this data, we recommend creating a subcategory of IBS, called "Atopic IBS", which would include patients with typical IBS who also have an extensive allergy history, including eczema (skin allergy), hay fever (allergy to common environmental allergens that presents as stuffy and runny nose and sneezing) and asthma.

❖ **What about "food allergy"? Is that also related to IBS?**

Dr. Farhadi: Technically speaking, these two are separate entities. However, some times it would be a diagnostic challenge to separate these two entities clearly. The hallmark of food allergy is an immediate or a consistent reaction to a particular food or class of foods. These reactions include swelling, pain and itching in the mouth and throat, abdominal pain and diarrhea just after ingestion of the particular food. These symptoms may or may not be associated with skin itching, rash, hives or shortness of breath. An extreme form of food allergy may present as anaphylaxis (a severe life threatening allergic response that requires urgent critical care and resuscitation). Occasionally, a food allergy may present with subtle or delayed symptoms, which makes the diagnosis of this disorder very difficult.

Dr. Tobin: It can be. With a food allergy the abdominal pain or discomfort can be accompanied by itching of the lips, inside of the mouth, tongue or throat or can even cause swelling in these areas and make it hard to talk or swallow. Some people will report that they get an itchy nose, skin rash or hives with diarrhea. When a person has severe swelling, shortness of breath or dizziness, a person is said to have an "anaphylactic reaction" to that food and must completely avoid it and carry epinephrine for treatment. Allergic reactions to food usually occur within 2 hours of eating and will reoccur to some extent every time the food is eaten. In adults, the most common foods to cause reactions are peanuts, tree nuts, fish and shellfish. People who have seasonal allergies or a history of allergic eczema (skin rash) may have food reactions that are worse in the spring or fall like their seasonal allergies. They may have reactions to fruits and vegetables that share proteins with the pollen. A reaction of itching or swelling that is limited to the mouth is known as oral allergy syndrome. Again, skin itching, diarrhea or even problems with shortness of breath can accompany oral symptoms with specific foods. These allergies may be harder to identify but a food diary with the time of onset after eating and symptoms, is an important first step to evaluating the role of food allergy with IBS. Some foods that commonly cause reactions in this way include apples, carrots, bananas, melons, cantaloupe, tree nuts and tomatoes.

❖ **I cannot tolerate milk. Each time I drink milk, I have bloating and diarrhea. Is this a milk allergy?**

Dr. Tobin: This is not a milk allergy. This reaction is typical for lactose intolerance. This is caused by not having the enzyme or protein to break down the milk protein. Sometimes using products with the enzyme lactase added, will allow you to have milk without symptoms. Lactose intolerance is usually seen in families of Mediterranean ancestry but can also occur after a severe infection of the bowel and as people age.

❖ **I have not had a trip abroad, or had any recent changes in my environment, such as diet or stress. Nevertheless, I have diarrhea, which began gradually over a period of 6 months. Is there any subgroup of IBS that I belong to?**

The other new development in the field of IBS regards an imbalance in cytokines among IBS patients.[16, 23, 29] As you may remember, cytokines are the chemicals that are released by various cells, particularly immune and Mast cells, and mediate inflammatory changes in the body. There are pro-inflammatory and anti-inflammatory cytokines in the body. The imbalance between the cytokines in IBS is in favor of the predominance of pro-inflammatory over anti-inflammatory cytokines. This imbalance in IBS points toward a mild subclinical (not clinically overt) inflammatory process that cannot be detected by our conventional diagnostic methods, such as endoscopy or tissue biopsy (microscopic exam). Again, this is a new finding in a subgroup of patients with diarrhea-predominant IBS and does not apply to all IBS patients. The relevance and therapeutic application of this finding to IBS has yet to be determined.

❖   **So, it seems that there are several subclasses of IBS: post-infectious, post-stress, atopic ...This is very confusing!**

Well, that is true in some sense. These subclasses are not considered formal classification categories in IBS. I believe that IBS is a presentation of different "diseases", all of which share one thing in common: "dysmotility-hypersensitivity" of the intestines. However, our limited current knowledge does not permit us to tease out these diseases from each other and thus, we clump all of these diseases together under a unifying umbrella of "IBS". As a result, our current classification of IBS is based on the type of bowel habit. Using this classification, we divide IBS into three types: diarrhea-predominant, constipation-predominant and mixed diarrhea-constipation.

Chapter 3

SYMPTOMS
(COMPLAINTS)

In this chapter, you will learn:

✓   _What the symptoms of IBS are._

✓   _Why abdominal pain is usually triggered by food._

✓   _Whether weight loss and loss of appetite are symptoms of IBS._

✓   _What the natural course of IBS is._

✓   _What's going to happen to you._

✓   _Whether smoking is a stimulant._

✓   _What the source of so much gas is._

✓   _How lactose intolerance could create symptoms similar to IBS._

❖ **What are the symptoms of IBS?**

Figure 9: Common symptoms associated with IBS

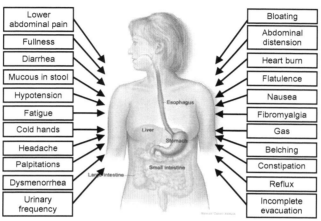

At first glance, the symptoms of IBS may seem to be limited to the gastrointestinal tract. However, there are numerous symptoms outside of the GI tract that are also associated with IBS "see Figure 9." These extra-intestinal symptoms are mainly related to an underlying generalized anxiety. As you see in the picture, IBS symptoms include a wide range of complaints such as abdominal pain, cramps, bloating, fullness, abdominal distension, constipation, incomplete bowel evacuation, flatulence, nausea and belching. Extra-intestinal IBS symptoms include headaches, palpitations, frequent urination (urinary frequency), painful menstruation (dysmenorrhea) and cold hands. IBS is also commonly associated with diffuse muscular pain (fibromyalgia) and chronic fatigue syndrome (sense of lack of energy and tiredness all the time).

❖ **Are all of these symptoms present in all patients?**

No. Most IBS patients present with only a few of these symptoms.

❖   **How would you describe abdominal pain in IBS?**

Abdominal pain in IBS can present in different ways and the quality and frequency of the pain can change from time to time. Typically, abdominal pain in IBS is a crampy pain that occurs in the lower left part of the abdomen and usually improves with a bowel movement. In addition, the pain may be dull pain that is triggered by eating and occurs around the belly button (periumbilical area). It also may be experienced as burning, hunger pain in the upper abdomen. The site of the pain may change from time to time. It also can be experienced as a fleeting, tense, stabbing pain that occurs in the lower abdomen or rectum.

❖   **Why abdominal pain is usually triggered by food, and relieved by a bowel movement?**

Good question! It is not surprising that GI functional disorders show itself when the GI tract is functioning. An analogy would be a problem with your car engine that is only evident when your car engine is on. Obviously, food intake increases the activity of the gut via distention of stomach. This results in activity of BGA and release of hormones, all of which cause the GI tract to over-react in terms of motility and sensitivity. The relief of symptoms after bowel movement is mainly due to relief of the pressure that has been built up in the colon due to colonic distention.

❖   **How come the symptoms are not always present?**

Why do I have them only once in while?

The symptoms of IBS are the result of, or a reaction to, one or more stimuli. For example, imagine you are under a significant amount of stress, due to your new business. You may experience severe problems with eating certain food while you are under stress. However, you may be able to enjoy the same food without any problems during your vacation. Thus, the presentation of symptoms can change from time to time.

❖   **Is the response to different stimuli the same?**

No. As mentioned above, there is a wide spectrum of symptoms in this disease. On one end of the spectrum are those symptoms that are the result of intestinal hypersensitivity, such as abdominal pain. On the other end are symptoms, which result from intestinal dysmotility, such as diarrhea and constipation. There are only a minority of either IBS patients whose symptoms are at one or another end of this spectrum and present with only pain or motility problems. Most IBS patients have symptoms that fall in the middle of the spectrum such as cramps, fullness and distension. It is not surprising that you may have multiple symptoms that fall all along this spectrum.

❖   **Are weight loss and loss of appetite symptoms of IBS?**

No. These symptoms are red flags and are almost always signs of an organic disorder. One characteristic of IBS is maintaining a steady weight over time. In fact, any indication of weight loss, loss of appetite, fever, anemia or blood in the stool is not part of the IBS presentation and should be seriously investigated.

❖   **What is the natural course of IBS? What's gonna happen to me?**

This disorder is typically a chronic condition with intermittent symptoms. In other words, IBS may disturb you for some period of time and then go away for a few days, weeks or months, after which the cycle starts all over again. The length of time that symptoms persist depends on the presence of stimuli and could vary.

❖   **Does this mean that I am going to have my problem forever?**

Unfortunately, yes. This is why patients with IBS have been seen and treated by so many doctors. Perhaps one day we will find the etiology and a cure for IBS.

❖   **So, it's less likely that I will have a long-term disease-free interval. Is there any chance of complete remission?**

Although chances are slim, complete remission is still possible. Each year, a small minority of patients achieve complete remission, so there is certainly some reason to be optimistic.

❖   **What kind of food is considered a stimulant?**

Well, it is very difficult to answer this question. Food affects individuals differently. For example, soda produces bloating and dyspepsia in some, while relieving dyspepsia in others. Fresh fruit and vegetables cause discomfort in some individuals, while the majority of patients do not have any problems with this type of food. Therefore, defining a stimulant food for you is neither feasible nor practical. There is no rule of thumb that spices are stimulants or white bread is a non-stimulant. The rule of "one size fits all" doesn't apply here. In fact, the definition of stimulant food is based solely on the individual's personal experiences.

❖ **So, you are telling me that food is not a stimulant per se, and certain foods are stimulants for only some people some of the time.**

Absolutely yes. It seems that you've got the point.

❖ **I realize now that we cannot exactly determine which food is a stimulant for all IBS patients. Could you at least tell me what kind of food is typically a stimulant?**

Pickles, especially garlic pickles, raw or fried garlic sauce, raw onions, spices and red or black peppers are usually the major stimulants. Also, ham, sausage, pizza, soda, as well as foods that contain sauces and marinades could be potent stimulants. Vegetable soup, greasy food and deep fried food are also common stimulants. Some, but not most, individuals cannot tolerate liquid foods, like soup, broth or gravy. Also, some individuals cannot tolerate fresh fruit, such as watermelon, cantaloupe, avocados, nectarines and tangerines. A few patients have problem with vegetables, like turnips, tomatoes, watercress or mixed spring greens.

❖ **Is a food stimulus necessary for the occurrence of symptoms?**

No. Symptoms can happen without any relation to food

intake.

❖ **What about smoking. Is it a stimulant?**

Smoking causes numerous pulmonary and extra-pulmonary problems. By increasing gastroesophageal reflux disease, and decreasing gastric mucosal defenses, smoking plays a significant role in causing peptic ulcer disease and dyspepsia. However, smoking is not considered a major stimulant in IBS.

❖ **What about alcoholic beverages? Is alcohol a stimulant?**

The effect of alcohol on the GI tract is significant and varies depending on a number of factors such as drinking history, type of drinking (i.e., beer, hard liquor, etc.) and amount consumed. Consumption of a large amount of alcohol could cause mucosal damage and abnormal intestinal motility, which might in turn aggravate the underlying dysmotility of the GI tract in people with IBS. However, the stress-reducing effects of alcohol might actually mitigate some of its irritating effects, thereby temporarily improving some IBS symptoms. Indeed, most alcoholics have problems with their GI motility and suffer from GI symptoms, which are directly or indirectly related to chronic alcohol abuse.

❖ **So do psychological stimuli play a major role in this type of situation?**

Usually, yes. However, there are some instances when you will not find any obvious psychological stimuli that are associated with your symptoms. Thus, you may experience symptoms related to dysmotility or bowel hypersensitivity without any obvious precipitating psychological cause.

❖ **Could you describe the diarrhea that is associated with IBS?**

The exact definition of diarrhea has always been a topic for discussion. Many parameters, such as ethnicity, culture and diet play an important role in the actual frequency and our expectation of the number and consistency of our bowel movements. In fact, the frequency of bowel movements varies widely from individual to individual. For example, some individuals may have three bowel movements a week, while others have three bowel movements a day and both situations could be considered normal, depending on the person's usual bowel function. For example, in many South American countries, normal bowel habits consist of two to three bowel movements per day; and individuals in these countries would think they were constipated if they had one bowel movement per day. There is also another classification for diarrhea that is based mainly on stool consistency and called Bristol Stool Form Scale or Bristol Stool Chart. In this classification, the appearance of the stool in a toilet has been categorized into seven groups. This classification was developed by Dr. K. W. Heaton at the University of Bristol and was first published in 1990.[30] Based on this scale the diarrhea stool starts from soft bleb with clear edges (Type 5) to fluffy pieces with ragged edges or mushy stool (Type 6) to extreme form of watery stool with no solid pieces (Type 7).

To return to your question, my definition is based on

both parameters and I think diarrhea is any significant increases in stool frequency or changes in stool consistency compared to the person's baseline bowel habits. You should also bear in mind that there are numerous reasons for diarrhea and IBS is only one of them. Other causes include lactose intolerance, parasitic infection, food allergy and other food-related problems. Among patients with IBS, diarrhea usually occurs in the morning; it is associated with increased mucus or whitish phlegm, with or without a significant amount of gas. Usually, people with this type of diarrhea describe their stool as initially soft or normal, followed by mushy or liquid stool. They usually go to the bathroom two to three times within a very brief period, due to a sense of incomplete evacuation. The frequency of the bowel movement is often no more than three to four times a day and sometimes it is interspersed with episodes of constipation. Nocturnal diarrhea that awakens the individual is not a symptom of IBS. However, if the patient suffers from insomnia and wakes up in the middle of the night for other reasons, it is not uncommon to have nocturnal bowel movements. Blood in the stool, bulky or greasy stool or weight loss are not associated with IBS. These are red flags for organic GI disorders and you should seek your doctor advice for these problems.

❖ **Could you describe the constipation that is associated with IBS?**

The definition of constipation is even more controversial than that of diarrhea. As I mentioned, the frequency of a bowel movement may vary from three times a week to three times a day in healthy individuals. Many physicians would consider less than three bowel movements per week to be constipation. Some physicians use Bristol Stool Chart for the definition of constipation. [30] Based on this scale the normal stool is either a soft sausage (Type 4) or a sausage with crack on it (Type 3). Harder stools that form sausage with lumps (Type 2) or separate hard lumps like nuts (Type 1) are considered constipation. In my opinion, definition of constipation should be based on the specific individual's routine bowel habit. Any significant changes in bowel habits, including change in consistency or decreased frequency of stool or increased effort in bowel movements, should be considered constipation. Similar to diarrhea, there are numerous reasons for constipation and IBS is only one of them. Constipation in IBS is usually associated with episodes of abdominal pain, cramps, colic, bloating and flatulence. Furthermore, many IBS patients complain of a sense of incomplete evacuation (incomplete bowel movements, or the need to use the bathroom several times within a very short period of time). Pencil or palette-like stools are also common features. Some individuals have intermittent diarrhea and constipation.

❖ **I have constipation and each time I have to strain a lot. I do not have any abdominal pain or other symptoms. Do I have IBS?**

Dr. Drossman: Irritable bowel syndrome (IBS) is diagnosed when there is a combination of symptoms, specifically abdominal pain with usually diarrhea, constipation or at times, both.[13, 14] You say you have constipation, and if that is associated with pain, you may have IBS. If you don't have pain or if you have pain that is not associated with your constipation, you may have what is called functional constipation. People with symptoms of constipation who need to strain may do so for two possible reasons. The first is that when stools are very hard and in small pieces, it is difficult to expel the stool easily and often the person must strain to evacuate. Another possibility can be when the muscles in the pelvic floor don't relax properly. This is called pelvic floor dysfunction or pelvic floor dys-synergia.[13, 31] In this case, one of the pelvic floor muscle groups, called the puborectalis, remains tense when it should relax during defecation, and this keeps the passageway narrow and at an angle thus preventing stool from passing through the rectum. In fact, the more one strains, the more acute the angle and the more tense the muscle becomes. Your gastroenterologist can make this diagnosis with a rectal examination and a special procedure called anorectal motility. If present, the condition can be treated using a type of biofeedback that teaches you through exercises to relax this muscle and ultimately reduce the straining.[32]

❖ **How would you describe the abdominal pain in IBS?**

As I mentioned earlier, there is a considerable amount of variation in the type of abdominal pain in IBS. In the majority of cases, the pain is crampy and occurs in the lower part of the abdomen. Typically, it usually increases just before the bowel movement and gradually diminishes afterward. Pain experienced in the periumbilical (around umbilicus) and mid-upper abdomen are other common forms of abdominal pain in IBS. This type of pain is usually associated with fullness and bloating and increases with food consumption. Most patients experience some discomfort and food craving just before mealtime. This is in contrast to the sharp hunger pains that are observed among patients with peptic ulcers. Similarly, the pain that awakens patients in the middle of the night is fairly typical of peptic ulcers and not due to IBS. Yet other forms of abdominal pain, although uncommon, in IBS include pain that is not associated with food intake or bowel movements, abdominal pain that changes in location and quality from time to time, and atypical abdominal pain that moves to the back, rectum or urinary bladder.

❖   **What is the reason for distension and gas in IBS? What is the source of this much gas?**

Interestingly, feelings of bloating and fullness among patients with IBS are not essentially due to an increase in the gas content of the bowel!!! You may ask, "How could this be possible?" The bowels are in a state of mild but continuous contraction, which is called "tone". When the tone is increased, even the presence of small amounts of gas in the lumen of the bowel increases the pressure inside the bowel. This could be experienced as discomfort and misinterpreted as a significant amount of gas. The intestine of people with IBS is similar to a thick balloon, in which a minimal increase in air creates a lot of pressure. In contrast, large amounts of air in the normal bowel (similar to a thin balloon) create a minimal increase in pressure. Unfortunately, the release of some of the gas results in only minimal and transient relief. Several studies have indicated that the majority of IBS patients do not have significantly more luminal gas compared to healthy individuals. I should mention that in a minority of patients with IBS, the feeling of abdominal distension is associated with a *visible* distention or increase in abdominal size. Among these individuals, abnormal motility results in retention of luminal gas. A recent study of IBS subjects found that the passage of gas could be hampered in the GI tract due to poor motility. This results in the accumulation of gas in the bowel lumen due to a series of ineffective, back and forth movements of the bowel. This ineffective handling of gas by the GI tract results in a buildup of gas in the bowel and a sense of bloating.[33] Other possible causes for distention and gas are lactose intolerance, bacterial overgrowth and aerophagia. Aerophagia is the swallowing of air and usually happens during stressful situations or rushed eating. I will discuss bacterial overgrowth and lactose intolerance later in this chapter. I also should mention that there are a variety of foods that inherently produce a large amount of gas such as beans, legumes and certain vegetables such as turnips and beets.

❖ **How could lactose intolerance create similar symptoms?**

As mentioned above, lactase deficiency, or lactose intolerance, is another disorder that must be seriously considered when thinking about the diagnosis of IBS. Indeed, lactose intolerance can be easily confused with IBS. "Lactase" is an enzyme in the proximal part of the small intestine that digests the milk sugar "lactose". The intestines of babies typically have a strong capacity to digest this milk sugar. As we get older, the amount and capability of this enzyme declines. This process occurs more quickly in some ethnic groups such as African-Americans and Asians. These problems are especially likely to occur when a large amount of this type of sugar is consumed. Undigested sugar will rush into the large bowel, where it will be consumed by bacteria producing several gases. One such gas is hydrogen, which is used to diagnose bacterial overgrowth using a Breath Test. Symptoms of IBS are common among people with lactose intolerance, particularly distension and gas following consumption of dairy products.

❖ **What is bacterial overgrowth? As you said, we normally have a ton of bacteria in our bowel, right?**

Yes, we have a large number of bacteria in the mouth and large bowel. Due to the acidic environment of the stomach as well as the digestive enzymes in the small bowel, the environment of the stomach and the small bowel are almost germ-free. In some instances, this germ-free environment becomes populated with bacteria, which competes with the host (human) to acquire nutritious materials that are supposed to be absorbed across the wall of the small bowel. The bacteria also make a variety of toxins and irritants that can result in bowel inflammation and irritation, creating symptoms of diarrhea, bloating and abdominal pain. This condition is called bacterial overgrowth. Recently, there was a report claiming that a significant group of IBS patients have bacterial overgrowth as the cause of their symptoms.[34] However, more recent reports were not able to duplicate this finding.[35, 36]

❖ **Is nausea a common symptom in IBS?**

Nausea is not common in IBS; however, it is not uncommon in patients with non-ulcer dyspepsia. As mentioned above, non-ulcer dyspepsia is another type of functional bowel disorders that is frequently associated with IBS. Nausea is due to backward peristalsis of the stomach and proximal small intestine (duodenum). Thus, there may be a backflow of bile into the stomach. If nausea occurs in IBS, it is usually short-lived in the morning or at mealtime and diminishes temporarily with food. Vomiting, however, is associated with strong contractions of the stomach and abdominal wall muscles and rarely occurs in functional bowel disorders including IBS.

❖   **You mentioned that sometimes there are extra-intestinal symptoms. What are they?**

Although most of the symptoms of IBS are limited to the GI tract, footprints of IBS can be detected in other organ systems of the body. These symptoms are not part of IBS or functional bowel disease per se, but are frequently associated with these disorders. For example, urinary frequency, fatigue, panic attacks, episodes of orthostasis (dizziness while standing), migraine and tension headaches, dysmenorrhea (painful menstruation), palpitations and cold, clammy hands are frequent complaints among IBS patients and may be related to underlying stress and anxiety.

❖   **Does heredity play any role in this disorder?**

As I explained earlier, the problem in IBS is in the heightened activity of the Brain-Gut Axis. There are some reports of clusters of IBS patients within the same family, but the exact role of hereditary factors in IBS is not clear. It seems that the presence of one family member with IBS increases the risk of IBS among other family members, thus suggesting a role for genetic factors. However, this also may be due to common environmental factors shared by the same family members, such as food, psychological factors or even exposure to infectious agents, including post-infectious IBS. It was not long ago when we thought that heredity played a significant role in peptic ulcers. Now we know that the cluster of peptic ulcers in a family is due to the exposure of multiple family members to the same bacteria.

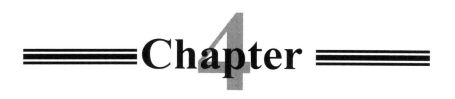

Chapter 4

DIAGNOSIS
(DISEASE IDENTIFICATION)

In this chapter, you will learn:

✓   *How we diagnose IBS.*

✓   *Whether there is any specific test that can diagnose IBS.*

✓   *Why you should have endoscopies, X-rays and CT scans, if these tests are "normal".*

✓   *Why you should repeat lab tests every couple of months, if these tests are normal.*

✓   *Whether everyone with IBS should be tested for lactose intolerance.*

✓   *What the role of bacterial overgrowth is in IBS.*

❖ **How do you diagnose this disorder?**

Figure 10: Commonly used diagnostic tests in IBS

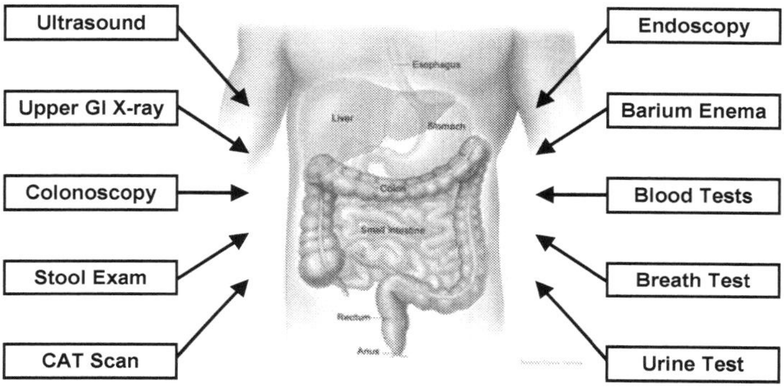

One of the major concerns in this disorder is arriving at an accurate diagnosis. In the majority of cases, the diagnosis is made based on a detailed patient history and a thorough physical examination. Rome Criteria is a diagnostic framework that should be used in all clinical setting and its use eliminates the need for many unnecessary diagnostic studies. "see Figure 10." Occasionally, some tests are required to rule out organic GI disorders or other potential diagnoses.

❖ **Is there any specific test that can diagnose IBS?**

Unfortunately, no. The tests enable us to exclude other diagnoses such as celiac disease and inflammatory bowel disease (IBD) which includes Crohn's Disease and Ulcerative Colitis, or other organic GI disorders. IBS is a clinical diagnosis, which means that self-reported symptoms are the mainstay of the diagnosis.

❖ **If endoscopies, X-rays and CT scans are "normal" in**

IBS, why should I have these tests?

To diagnose IBS, there is no need to perform all of these tests. However, in some cases, symptoms of other organic GI diseases such as inflammatory bowel disease and celiac disease, or disorders of other organs in the abdominal cavity such as liver, uterus, ovaries and kidneys are very similar to IBS. Thus, in order to exclude other diagnoses, it may be necessary to do endoscopies, X-rays, CT scans, ultrasounds, blood tests and Breath Tests.

❖ **What is the role of blood, urine and stool tests?**

Again, these tests are ways to exclude organic GI disorders. For example, the results of a stool test can detect an intestinal parasite while the presence of microscopic blood in the stool may suggest the presence of colon cancer, polyps or ulcers. Stool tests also can be used for diagnosis of pancreatic insufficiency. Blood tests can detect anemia as a sign of organic GI disorders. Data from blood tests also can help in the diagnosis of malabsorption, inflammatory bowel disease and celiac disease. Nowadays, we also can perform some genetic tests for celiac disease using blood samples. Urine tests might indicate a possible urinary tract infection or presence of a kidney stone. Usually, IBS patients undergo a battery of these tests and most of the time, the results are normal.

❖ **If these lab tests are normal, why do the doctors repeat them every couple of months?**

Many physicians believe that the best approach for diagnosing IBS is by monitoring the patient over a period of time with periodic clinical exams and simple lab tests. This will rule out the possibility of an organic GI problem and lead to an early detection of abnormalities.

❖ **What is the specific purpose of performing a barium enema, colonoscopy or endoscopy? And, when are these tests indicated?**

An upper endoscopy, which scans the esophagus, stomach and duodenum, is helpful for diagnosing upper GI disorders, such as a peptic ulcer, reflux esophagitis, and gastritis. Additionally, a tissue biopsy at the time of an upper endoscopy can be used for diagnosis of gastritis caused by Helicobacter infection and/or celiac disease. An upper endoscopy with the use of ultrasonic devices (endoscopic ultrasound) may be used to diagnose diseases of the biliary tract (including gallstones) and/or the pancreas (such as chronic pancreatitis). A colonoscopy can be used to diagnose inflammatory bowel disease, colonic polyps or colon cancer. Barium enema is alternative to colonoscopy. Virtual colonoscopy or CT colography is a type of CT scan of the colon and is a newer technique in which the colon image is reconstructed into a three-dimensional picture and can be used to visualize colonic abnormalities. Indications for an upper endoscopy include upper abdominal pain, fullness, diarrhea and distension. The indication for colonoscopy however, is lower abdominal pain, diarrhea or blood in the stool.

❖ **What is SmartPill® Gastrointestinal (GI) Monitoring System and does it have any role in IBS?**

The SmartPill® Gastrointestinal (GI) Monitoring System

is an ingestible capsule, which measures pressure, acidity, and temperature as it travels through gastrointestinal tract. This information is transferred through wireless technology to a data receiver outside of the body and the data is recorded for evaluation by doctors. This information could be used to assess the gastric and intestinal motility, pH and temperature. This capsule is a single-use device and is excreted naturally from the body, usually within a day or two. The data receiver should be worn on a belt clip or a lanyard around the patient's neck. In addition, the data receiver may be removed for sleeping or taking showers but should be kept within 5 feet of the patient. Currently the SmartPill® GI monitoring system has been only approved for evaluation of disturbed stomach motility (gastroparesis). However, the information obtained from this device may make it feasible to be used for evaluation of motility problem of other parts of the GI tract and particularly IBS.

❖   **I have heard that there is camera that can show the entire gastrointestinal system. Should I get this test as part of work-up for IBS?**

Pillcam ® is a very small camera that can fit into a pill size capsule and can record images of the entire stomach and the small bowel. The Pillcam® is ingested similar to a regular pill. The name of this test is Video Capsule Endoscopy and is currently being performed in many centers throughout the world. The camera inside the capsule is equipped with a light source that will be used to illuminate the inside of the bowel during the image capture. The images that are captured by the camera will be transmitted through a wireless technology to a small pager like device that is worn around your belt. Thus, there is no need to retrieve the capsule to obtain the images. The Pillcam® capsule is disposable and the battery inside the capsule wears out after a few hours of use. The Pillcam® capsule records 2 images per second for 8 hours continuously producing 50,000 images. After completion of the test (8 hours), the images will be downloaded from the device into the physician's desktop computer for viewing. Playing these images on the computer creates a near continuous motion picture like a movie. This procedure does not require prior bowel cleansing or preparation and during the test, you can go back to your daily routine. In addition, this test is painless and minimally invasive with very few complications. However, there are some limitations to this test. First of all this test is only designed to diagnose lesions in the stomach and small bowel. This is because the large bowel always contains fecal material and the test is done without any pre-procedure bowel cleansing. Additionally, there is no way to control the camera's views or speed of passage through various parts of the GI tracts. Therefore, there could be a great variation in the speed of the passage and recording of the images by the camera. Lastly, the lack of therapeutic capabilities on the device can mandate further endoscopic intervention for obtaining tissue samples or treatment of the lesions. Overall, this useful test is becoming increasingly popular because of the ease of use and minimal invasiveness. The test is currently being used to diagnose several gastrointestinal disorders including celiac disease, small bowel Crohn's disease and benign or malignant tumors of the small bowel. This is particularly important because this part of the bowel is less accessible to conventional endoscopic examinations. Currently, this test is not indicated routinely in patients with IBS. However, those with chronic abdominal pain in whom the diagnosis of small bowel Crohn's disease or celiac disease are likely to benefit from this test.

❖ **A friend of mine had a special CT scan named CT-Entroclysis for his abdominal pain. What is this test? Is it different from usual CT scan?**

CT scan or CAT scan of the abdomen provides a three dimensional image of the abdominal cavity using x-ray beams. This imaging technique makes it possible to see the details of the organs inside the abdominal cavity, which include the gastrointestinal tract. For better delineation of the gastrointestinal tract, this test is being performed after ingestion of an oral contrast agent. Due to the long length of the small bowel, usually the oral contrast is not distributed well all over the small bowel. Thus, subtle and small abnormalities in the small bowel could have been easily missed. Recently, the radiologist came up with the new idea of using a large amount of very dilute oral contrast to further improve the quality of the small bowel imaging. Using this newer technique, it is possible to perform abdominal CT scan and a dedicated small bowel x-ray study at the same time (two birds with one stone). This test is the preferred method for investigation of abdominal pain in some centers. However, it needs a special oral contract, a dedicated CT technician and a radiologist familiar with this test. Thus, this test is only being performed in a limited number of medical centers.

❖ **What tests are available for finding food allergies?**

Dr. Tobin: When trying to see if there is a food allergy, it is important to keep a diary, which describes the food, the time of symptoms after eating the food and if any other allergy symptoms came at the same time like a runny nose, hives, skin rash, shortness of breath or swelling. Skin testing can be done with food extracts at the allergist office or the allergist may ask you to bring the food that you are having problems with and skin test you with the fresh food. Based on the results you and your doctor may decide on an elimination diet of the food and then restarting it. If there is a question, you might have a food challenge in the allergists' office.

If your reaction to food caused severe symptoms, your blood may be drawn looking for the allergy antibody to the food. Based on these results, further skin testing or oral challenges may be done in the allergists' office. Currently, other antibody tests against food proteins are being studied to see if they might be helpful for finding problem foods in patients with IBS.

❖ **Is psychological evaluation a necessary tool for the diagnosis of IBS?**

Psychological evaluation is not necessary, but can be a useful tool in the evaluation and management of IBS. In many instances, a psychologist could be extremely helpful in evaluating underlying psychological problems, establishing coping strategies through cognitive behavioral therapy and teaching various relaxation methods.

❖ **While other doctors suggested several diagnostic tests, you based your diagnosis on clinical grounds. Why is there so much difference in doctors' approaches to this disorder?**

As I mentioned earlier, diagnosis of IBS is primarily based on the clinical judgment of an experienced physician. The results of certain tests can be helpful for excluding other possible diagnoses. In some circumstances, the diagnosis is obvious, or the patient has a prior medical workup that makes it quiet easy to establish the diagnosis of IBS without any additional tests. However, sometimes this diagnosis can only be reached after an exhaustive battery of tests. In the meantime, it is important to acknowledge that the differences in physicians' experience can critically affect the way they approach their patients' problems.

❖ **I was diagnosed with IBS 8 years ago. Now, my doctor is telling me I have celiac disease. How could this be possible?**

Good question. Although this is not a common scenario, it could happen. The diagnosis of some diseases, particularly celiac disease, has changed dramatically over the last decade. In fact, the results of many tissue biopsies that were taken years ago and were reported as normal could have actually been interpreted as early celiac disease by today's standards. In addition, there are many new lab tests or genetic markers, which make it possible to diagnose celiac disease very early on, in the preclinical stages (even before the presence of clinical symptoms). It is also important to note that the symptoms of celiac disease can be very similar to IBS. This is why I mentioned earlier that to reach an accurate diagnosis of IBS, it is appropriate to monitor patients for an extended period of time.

❖ **What is celiac disease?**

Celiac disease is due to hypersensitivity to gluten in wheat or bran in bread, cookies, cake and many other foods. The spectrum of symptoms of celiac disease ranges from gastrointestinal symptoms such as abdominal pain, diarrhea, constipation and bloating, to non-GI symptoms, including a change in mood, iron deficiency anemia, repeated fracture due to osteoporosis, weight loss, and depression.

❖ **How do you diagnose celiac disease?**

In the past, the diagnosis of celiac disease was based on clinical symptoms, the presence of changes in the intestinal mucosa under the microscope (pathology) and reversal of clinical and pathological changes after the patient switches to a gluten-free diet. Currently, we also take advantage of blood tests to check for the presence of specific antibodies and genetic evaluation, for better diagnosis of this condition.

❖ **What is a lactose Breath Test? What does it diagnose?**

As mentioned above, the presence of lactase that breaks down the milk sugar, lactose is essential for digestion of milk and dairy products. When an individual with reduced ability to digest lactose consumes a large amount of dairy products, the enzyme is easily overwhelmed. As a result, the undigested sugar travels through the small intestine and reaches the large bowel, where bacteria consumes the sugar and produces a significant amount of gases, including hydrogen. Hydrogen is an odorless gas that is absorbed in the blood stream and is eventually excreted through the lungs in our exhaled breath. During a Breath Test, the patient is provided with a standard amount of lactose and after a certain period of time, the amount of hydrogen in his/her breath is measured. If this amount is high, it means that there is not enough lactase in the intestine and the patient has lactase deficiency, or lactose intolerance.

❖   **So, should every one with IBS be tested for lactose intolerance?**

Although the lactose Breath Test is a standard method for the diagnosis of lactase deficiency, the most practical approach toward diagnosis of lactose intolerance is based on one's response to the elimination of milk and dairy products from the diet. In other words, if most or all of the symptoms reduced as a result of a dairy-free diet, there is a strong possibility that lactase deficiency is causing the problems. Furthermore, a hydrogen Breath Test is not sensitive enough to detect lactase deficiency in all cases. Thus, I recommend that any patient with IBS should undergo a lactose-free trial diet for at least 2-4 weeks.

❖   **Is there another type of Breath Test?**

Yes. Another useful Breath Test is the Lactulose Breath Test, which can be used to diagnose bacterial overgrowth.

❖   **How does a Breath Test diagnose bacterial overgrowth?**

As I mentioned before, bacterial overgrowth is the accumulation of bacteria in parts of the GI tract that are normally free of any germs. One such place is the small bowel. The gold-standard method of diagnosing bacterial overgrowth is by taking a tiny amount of small bowel fluid and culturing this fluid in order to detect the number and type of any bacteria that are present. If the amount of germs found within this fluid exceeds a set limit, bacterial overgrowth is diagnosed. However, this method is cumbersome and has been replaced largely by either the Lactulose Breath Test or antibiotic trial therapy. In the

Lactulose Breath Test, a large amount of Lactulose (do not confuse this term with milk sugar or lactose) is given to the patient orally. Since the human GI tract is devoid of any enzymes to break down Lactulose, this sugar escapes digestion and absorption in the human intestine. Instead, it travels down the small bowel intact until it reaches the colon where it is digested by colonic bacteria. The digestion by bacteria results in the release of hydrogen gas in the bowel, which is absorbed in the blood. Similar to the lactose Breath Test, hydrogen will be excreted in the exhaled breath and the amount of this gas is measured in the collected exhaled breath in a bag. In a normal situation, the increase in the amount of hydrogen gas in the exhaled breath takes about a couple hours. This corresponds to the travel time of the sugar through the small bowel. In the case of bacterial overgrowth, the bacteria in the small bowel digest the Lactulose and release the hydrogen gas while the sugar is still in the small bowel. In this case, we would see an earlier rise in breath hydrogen, after less than an hour of the consumption of a load of Lactulose. Such an observation is diagnostic for this condition.

❖   **Is bacterial overgrowth common in IBS?**

Over the past decade, there has been an increase in the amount of information regarding the prevalence of bacterial overgrowth among patients with IBS. In one study, the authors claimed that up to 80% of IBS subjects had this condition and responded well to antibiotic treatment.[34] However, the results of this research have not been replicated by other scientists.[35, 36] In general, I think that bacterial overgrowth should be considered as part of the differential diagnosis of IBS and should be investigated in the subgroup of patients who present with diarrhea, bloating and abdominal pain.

❖   **I have abdominal pain, diarrhea and bloating only when I eat coconut or hazel nuts. Otherwise, I have no problems with food. Do I have IBS?**

Your symptoms are more likely due to a food allergy rather than IBS. Food allergies and food intolerance also can be easily confused with IBS. In these situations, an individual usually has GI symptoms only when he/she is exposed to a specific food. Food allergies or food intolerance usually first occur in childhood, while IBS typically presents later in life. In addition, the response to a specific food is typically identical in a food allergy and food tolerance. In contrast, in IBS, the response can be quite variable, and at times, individuals do not develop symptoms at all. Additionally, in patients with IBS, the symptoms are usually not limited to one or two specific foods. That being said, there are some cases when the distinction between a food allergy and IBS is blurred. In fact, some people have a combination of both conditions.

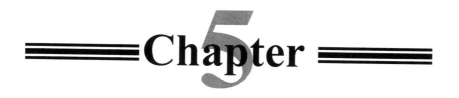 **Chapter 5**

TREATMENT
(HOW TO DEAL WITH IBS)

In this chapter, you will learn:

✓   _Whether there is any treatment for IBS._

✓   _What these treatments are._

✓   _Whether these treatments are effective._

✓   _Whether you should get a psychological or psychiatric evaluation._

✓   _What the commonly used alternative medicine are in IBS._

❖ **Is there any treatment for this disorder?**

Figure 11: Commonly used treatments in IBS

Proton pump inhibitors	Tums, Antacid
Anxiolytics	Psychotherapy
Antidepressant	Spasmolytics
GasX, Simethicon	Relaxation therapy
Herbal medicine	Dietary restrictions
Hypnosis	Acupuncture
Homeopathy	Meditation

Yes. There are several options for the treatments for IBS "see Figure 11."

❖ **Are these treatment options effective?**

When there are several options for treatment of a particular disease, you can safely assume that none one of the options is ideal. If there was an ideal treatment for this condition, there would be no need for alternatives. That being said, there are many treatments that significantly reduce symptoms.

❖ **What are the current IBS treatments?**

There is no cure for this illness. The remedies, therefore, are geared toward the relief of symptoms. Treatments decrease stimuli, increase the sensory threshold in response to the stimuli, or offset the effects of stimuli. The treatment modalities include conventional medicine, dietary restriction, behavioral and psychological approaches, relaxation therapy, meditation, hypnosis, herbal remedies, homeopathy and other alternative medicine.

❖ **So, you're telling me that the benefit of these pills and medicines are just temporary.**

Yes. However, since IBS is periodic in nature, these treatment modalities could actually alleviate your symptoms for a reasonable period of time.

❖ **During the 5 years of my illness, I have tried many pills and medications. Nothing was effective. I am frustrated. Is there any hope for successful treatment?**

Yes. You are at a pivotal moment in the path of a successful treatment. How?!?!? A proper understanding of the nature of IBS is the main foundation of a successful IBS treatment. The basic elements of treatment include recognition and elimination of the contributing stimuli. It is also helpful to use appropriate therapies to offset the effect of these stimuli.

❖ **What do you mean by decreasing stimuli?**

As I explained earlier, certain stimuli trigger intestinal dysmotility or hypersensitivity. Thus, it is crucial to identify these stimuli and attempt to avoid them or decrease exposure to them. This approach primarily includes avoiding certain foods and managing stress, which are the major triggers for IBS flare-up

❖ **How can I reduce my stress if I cannot change my job, my work environment or my life style?**

Good question. As your question indicates, it can be very difficult to change one's job, work environment, social interactions and/or lifestyle. Although these changes are sometimes necessary, it is beyond the scope of this book. However, I encourage you to develop the skills necessary to

Figure 12: Breaking the vicious cycle of IBS

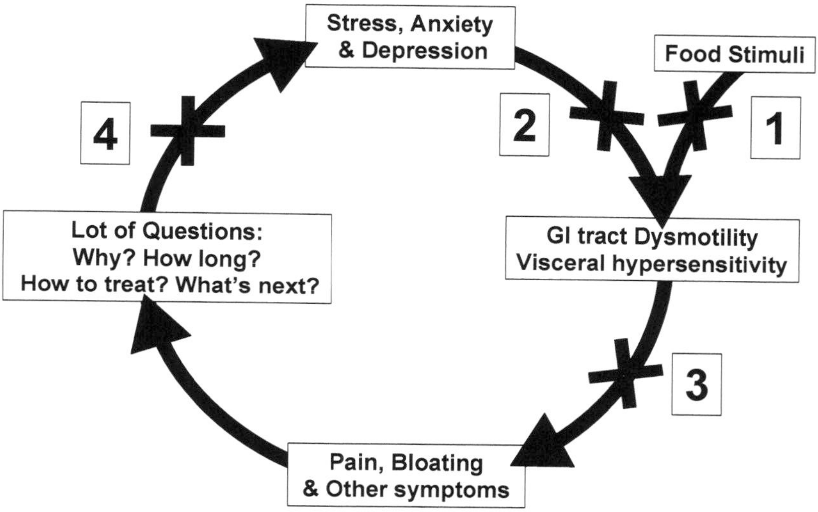

properly manage current levels of stress. I can not emphasize enough the importance of various technique specifically aimed at reducing stress as well as methods to manage the stress such as cognitive behavioral therapy that help you to change your reaction to stress. You can learn these techniques by visiting a psychologist, or other mental health professional who deal with stress management. These techniques have proven to be very successful among patients with a variety of physical health problems. As I mentioned above, you may not be able to completely eliminate the sources of stress in your life. But, you certainly are able to gain control over how you react to it. If you recall from the chapter on disease etiology, I discussed the vicious cycle of IBS and how stress serves as a major player in the cycle.

There are four potential targets for breaking this vicious cycle each of which can be approached by various therapeutic modalities "see Figure 12." The first two targets include the identification and avoidance of certain external stimuli, such as food and psychological factors. The third target lies in the therapeutic modalities, which alleviate symptoms. The fourth target is particularly important and involves education and reassurance. By properly understanding the nature and course of the illness, it is possible to reduce IBS-associated anxiety. As you can see, all of these approaches are geared toward interrupting the IBS cycle, which is the ultimate goal of successful treatment.

❖   **So, the reduction of IBS-induced stress and anxiety play a key role in my treatment.**

Absolutely!

❖   **What are the common ways that I can use to reduce my stress and anxiety?**

There are a growing numbers of stress management strategies. These treatment modalities include progressive muscle relaxation, meditation, yoga, music therapy, biofeedback, cognitive behavioral therapy, hypnotherapy (hypnosis), and dynamic psychotherapy. The majority of these interventions are designed to teach patients effective techniques that foster deep relaxation and reduce the daily tensions that increase stress and exacerbate IBS symptoms. Thus, it is not surprising that these interventions can successfully reduce symptoms of IBS.[37-40] Interestingly, research in this field also has indicated that the benefits of the majority of these interventions are sustained over a long period of time.[41-44]

❖ **Are these psychological treatments effective?**

The mechanisms through which these types of treatment work for patients are quite different from conventional biomedical treatments. Thus, the efficacy of psychological treatments is more difficult to evaluate by controlled trials. One of the major factors predicting the success of a particular therapeutic modality is the quality of the relationship between therapist and patient. Therefore, the success of these treatments varies substantially, depending on therapeutic rapport.[45] In general, these psychological interventions supplement medical treatment.

❖ **I've heard that IBS can be treated by hypnosis. Is that true?**

Dr. Jedel: Since current medical treatments do not alleviate all patients' symptoms of IBS, a number of alternative treatments are increasingly popular, particularly among those with chronic and severe symptoms. These treatments are typically used in conjunction with medical management and include cognitive-behavioral therapy, biofeedback, stress management and hypnosis. A number of research studies have shown that hypnosis can have a positive impact on gastrointestinal functioning as well as improving IBS symptoms. A typical course of hypnosis treatment spans 4 to 12 weekly or twice-monthly sessions, lasting about 30 minutes. During each session, patients participate in hypnosis, which is followed by deep relaxation exercises and the use of gut-directed guided imagery. Many hypnotherapists also provide patients with hypnosis CDs, which can be used throughout the week and upon conclusion of treatment. Although hypnosis has been successful in improving IBS-symptoms among numerous patients, researchers are not entirely clear on why it works. This important question continues to be investigated. What we do know, however, is that the brain and the gut are constantly communicating and influencing each other (this is referred to as the brain-gut axis). For example, when the mind confronts stressful events, anxiety and/or depression, symptoms of IBS can be triggered or exacerbated. The mind can also have a positive influence on gut functioning. Thus, when patients participate in hypnosis, and are in a deep state of relaxation and calm, their gastrointestinal tract may benefit as well.

❖ **Do you suggest a psychological or psychiatric evaluation for me?**

No, but let me explain. First, I want to clarify the difference between a psychological evaluation and a psychiatric evaluation. Psychological assessment is conducted by a psychologist and is geared toward understanding the patient's personality and psychological dynamics. This may help recognize any psychological symptoms, such as anxiety and depression that, although mild, still affect IBS symptoms. Psychologists also can assist by developing an appropriate treatment approach and choosing the types of interventions, such as stress management, that will ultimately help reduce IBS symptoms. Whether it is necessary to seek psychological evaluation for subtle psychological problems is a matter of debate. In contrast, there are a minority of IBS patients whose psychological symptoms (i.e. anxiety or depression) are severe enough to warrant a formal psychiatric evaluation. A psychiatric evaluation is conducted by a psychiatrist, who manages symptoms with medication, such as antidepressants. I do not suggest a routine psychiatric evaluation for IBS patients.

❖ **What is the role of fiber in IBS?**

Research has shown that fiber improves bowel movements by increasing the frequency and bulk of stool as well as decreasing the pressure inside the colon. The use of fiber supplements has been part of the standard management of IBS. However, data regarding the effect of fiber in IBS is conflicting. These findings may be due to differences in symptoms and type of fiber used in various studies. For example, wheat bran may decrease constipation by improving intestinal motility, while psyllium acts by improving stool consistency. Both are equally effective for relief of symptoms. Fiber works like a sponge. It works by holding and increasing the amount of water in the intestinal lumen. This softens the stool. Considering the "sponge" analogy, fiber would not be very effective in constipation unless it is used with adequate hydration. Interestingly, fiber helps IBS patients with diarrhea via the same mechanism as a sponge. Here, fiber absorbs the extra water in the intestinal lumen and changes a liquid stool into a soft one. Thus, fiber works in either constipation or diarrhea and helps the patient to have a formed and soft stool.

❖ **Everything I've heard about fiber is positive. Are**

there any disadvantages?

Yes. Fiber can cause bloating. Since fiber can be fermented by intestinal bacteria, it can result in production of an excess amount of gas. This problem is particularly troublesome when a large amount of fiber is introduced into the diet.

The good news is that bloating can be easily overcome by starting with a very low dose of fiber and *gradually* increasing the amount over a period of weeks rather than days. Typically, I recommend that patients begin with half a teaspoon of fiber twice a day and increase the amount gradually every few days until it results in a desired effect, which is 1 to 2 soft bowel movements per day.

❖   **Are there different types of fiber?**

As mentioned above, different kinds of fiber act through different mechanisms. Thus, the type of fiber you consume is of paramount importance. Individuals with constipation are more likely to benefit from psyllium or Metamucil, while bran powder is better suited for people with diarrhea.

❖   **I eat a lot of vegetables and fruits each day. Do I need a supplemental fiber pill?**

You should know that, although a fiber supplement such as fiber pills or powder is not superior to eating a fiber-rich diet such as vegetables and fruit, most people do not consume the required amount of fiber in their typical diet.

❖   **What kinds of medicines are used in IBS?**

Current treatment of IBS is based on symptom relief. The medications used for IBS improve intestinal dysmotility, intestinal hypersensitivity, or both. Medications that modify intestinal motility act by increasing peristalsis or decreasing spasms. These medications are called prokinetics or spasmolytics, respectively. Prokinetics and other laxatives are particularly helpful for relieving the symptoms of bloating and constipation, while spasmolytics relax intestinal contractions and are helpful in the management of abdominal pain and cramps. There are some motility agents, which reduce peristaltic activity and can be used to relieve diarrhea. Some medications act by modulating the perception of pain and thus improve patients' tolerance of pain. Some medications, such as anti-depressants and serotonin-like agents, are difficult to categorize into these groups since they have the ability to modify both intestinal motility and sensitivity.

❖ **What are commonly used prokinetic and laxative agents?**

Prokinetic agents are a group of medication which improves intestinal peristalsis and intestinal transit time.[46] Domperidone (Motilium®) is an example of a prokinetic agent that improves gastric emptying. It is effective for reducing bloating and abdominal pain after meals, particularly in non-ulcer dyspepsia. This medicine is not readily available in the United States and should be purchased from abroad. Cisapride (Propulsid®) is a medication that acts like serotonin and reduces constipation.[47] Due to a rare, but serious, cardiac side effect, this medication was recalled in the year 2000 by the Food and Drug Administration (FDA) and is no longer prescribed in the

U.S. Tegaserod (Zelnorm®), was another serotonin-like agent that was helpful for IBS patients with constipation, and also was recalled by the FDA due to its rare, though serious, cardiac side effects and it is now available under restricted use for treatment of IBS. Prokinetics are not the only group of medicine that improve the symptoms of bloating and constipation in IBS. Other laxatives can also be used for relieving these symptoms. This group of laxatives works by changing stool consistency. An example of this group of medicines is Amitiza® (Lubiprostone), which is a newer medicine that has been approved by the FDA for the treatment of IBS with constipation.

❖ **What are antidiarrheal agents?**

Antidiarrheal agents are helpful in the management of diarrhea and pain in IBS. Loperamide (Imodium®) and other antidiarrheal agents significantly decrease diarrhea and the sense of urgency in patients with IBS.[48] Loperamide is generally preferred to other opiates such as diphenoxylate (Lomotil®) because it does not directly affect the brain. Furthermore, diphenoxylate, when combined with anticholinergics (see below for description), may cause confusion, particularly in the elderly.[49] Cholestyramine (Questran®) is another antidiarrheal agent that has been used in IBS with variable success. The major disadvantage of Cholestyramine is its bad taste. Alosetron hydrochloride (Lotronex®) is a newer drug that blocks the effect of serotonin through type 3 serotonin receptors and retards small bowel and colonic transit in IBS.[50] This medicine is helpful for controlling diarrhea. It also affects intestinal sensation and improves abdominal pain.

❖ **What are spasmolytics or antispasmodics?**

Antispasmodics (also known as spasmolytics) are medications that are usually considered part of the "anticholinergic family". **What?!!** Anticholinergics are medications that block the effect of Vagus nerves on smooth muscle contraction. In other words, they relax smooth muscles. Antispasmodics are frequently prescribed for IBS patients with diarrhea and pain. Research has found that these agents were significantly more likely to reduce pain and to improve the patient's overall quality of life.[51] Commonly used spasmolytics are Dicyclomin (Bentyl®), Hyoscyamine (Anaspaz®, Levsin®, NuLev®, Levbid®), Metylscopalamin (Pamine®), Clidinium-C (Librax® is a combination of a spasmolytic, Hyoscyamine and an anxiolytic, Chlorodiazepoxide), Probanteline (Probantine ®), Symax (Duotab®). Despite similarities in their mechanism of action, there are differences in the onset of action and duration of action in these medications. Since these medications reduce bowel contractions, they can potentially result in constipation. Besides, the numerous potential side effects of anticholenergics and spasmolytics limit their popularity among physicians and patients.

Furthermore, these medications not only reduce contractions within the intestinal tract, they also reduce the contractions of the smooth muscle of other bodily organs. For example, reduction of contraction in the urinary bladder causes urinary retention. This is particularly concerting among those with an enlarged prostate. Relaxation of smooth muscles in the eyes results in temporary blurred vision. These medications also reduce secretion of salivary and lacrimal (tear) glands, which can result in, dry mouth and dry eyes. Drowsiness is another potential side effect of this group of medications. The newer versions of anticholinergic medications are expected to have fewer systemic side effects. Their effectiveness as well as complete side effect profile remains to be seen. There are also some herbal medications that have spasmolytic properties, such as spearmint and peppermint oil. These will be discussed below under the question regarding alternative medicine.

❖ **What are other medications that ease abdominal pain?**

Good question. The pain killers for IBS improve intestinal hypersensitivity by affecting the Brain-Gut Axis. In other words, they target serotonin receptors by either stimulating or inhibiting them. For example, Alosetron (Lotronex®) inhibits the type-3 serotonin receptors, while Tegaserode (Zelnorm®) stimulates type-4 serotonin receptors. Alosetron increases the thresholds for pain sensation, distension and urgency in subjects with IBS.[50] This medicine slows down the intestinal transit and improves the diarrhea in IBS.

Tegaserod not only improves motility in constipated subjects, it also increases the sensory threshold for pain and thus reduces abdominal pain in IBS.[52] As mentioned above, this medication is now available under restricted use. Prucalopride is similar to Tegaserod and its benefits are currently under active investigation.[53] Other groups of medicines that modify pain perception target the autonomic nervous system, which is a component of the brain-gut axis. Clonidine (Catapres®) affects receptors of the sympathetic nervous system and decreases painful colonic stimuli.[54] Octreotide (Sandostatin®) is another medicine that increases the sensory threshold for visceral pain and also slows GI motility in IBS.[55] Quite a few number of medications are currently under investigation for treatment of hypersensitivity and dysmotility in IBS and include SR-48,968, MEN-11,420,[56, 57] and brain-derived neurotrophic factor.[58]

❖ **What are psychotropic agents that are used in the treatment of IBS?**

Psychotropic medications are typically used to treat psychiatric symptoms, such as anxiety and depression. As I mentioned earlier, there are a number of patients with IBS who also have significant anxiety and depression. Obviously, these are the patients who can benefit from psychotropic medications.

❖ **I do not have any anxiety or depression but my doctor wrote me a prescription for an antidepressant!! Why did she do that?**

Besides their psychotropic effect, these medications can modify the brain-gut axis by affecting neurotransmitters along the axis and modifying the threshold for pain perception. The amount of the antidepressants that is required to effectively treat IBS is significantly less than what is used for the treatment of depression or anxiety.

❖ **What kind of antidepressant is most helpful in IBS?**

Almost all antidepressants have been prescribed to IBS patients, with variable degree of success. The most commonly used antidepressants are tricyclics and selective serotonin reuptake inhibitors (SSRIs) and Serotonin-norepinephrine reuptake inhibitors (SNRIs). The most commonly used tricyclics are Amitriptyline, Nortriptyline (Pamelor®), Imipramine (Tofranil®) and Doxepin (Sinequan®; Zonalon®). The beneficial effects of these medications are independent of their psychotropic effects.[59] The most commonly used SSRIs include Paroxetine (Paxil®) and Fluoxetine (Prozac®). The SNRIs are newer compared to the two mentioned above and the most commonly used SNRIs include Venlafaxine (Effexor®) and Duloxetine (Cymbalta®). Compared to tricyclics, SSRIs are less effective. However, they have fewer side effects compared to tricyclics and are also beneficial due to their anxiolytic properties. The SNRIs are also effective in the management of IBS.

❖ **What are the common herbal medicines in IBS? Are they effective and safe?**

Dr. Drossman: There are no scientifically established types of herbal medicines to treat IBS, though there may be many products available commercially. The use of herbal remedies is within the category of complementary or alternative medicine and can be used as long as they are not harmful, most often in addition to traditional treatments in western society. Many years ago, there was a study that showed greater benefit for individuals who had herbals selectively chosen by the herbalist. However, 10 years later it is still not clear whether there are standard herbal treatments for this condition.

Dr. Brown: Herbal medicines have been used for

centuries to treat functional bowel diseases. Recently Western literature has begun to publish studies of these treatments. One of the earliest studies was published in 1998 by a group from Australia. This was the first completed clinical trial concerning Chinese herbal medicine in the management of IBS published in non-Chinese literature. The researchers examined individual Chinese herbal medicines that were tailored to the patient's specific complaints, a mixture Chinese herbal medication for patients with functional bowel diseases regardless of their symptoms, and placebo medications. The mixture Chinese herbal medications contained up to 40 different herbs specifically selected by the herbalist to treat functional bowel disease. The 116 patients demonstrated a statistically superior benefit in overall symptom improvement for both the mixture and individualized Chinese herbal formulations compared to the placebo. There was no difference between the efficacy of the individual Chinese herbal medicine and the mixture formula. However, the duration of improvement was more durable lasting in the individualized medication. A more recent study from the Chinese University of Hong Kong, published in 2006, studied 119 patients who were randomized to receive either traditional Chinese medicine and or a placebo for the treatment of the their diarrhea-predominant IBS. The investigators in this trial examined global symptom improvement, a generalized assessment of the patient's overall well-being during the clinical trial. This is a very typical endpoint for many clinical trials completed in the field of functional bowel disease. This particular study did not show a difference in the responses between the patients in the placebo arm and those patients receiving the traditional Chinese medicine. The authors of this clinical trial concluded that Chinese herbal medicine was not effective in controlling the symptoms of diarrhea-predominant IBS. Tongxieyalfang (TXYF) is another Chinese herbal medicine that is used to manage IBS. In May 2006, the Journal of Alternative and Complementary Medicine published a study that reviewed the literature identifying randomized and controlled trials of this Chinese herbal medicine in the treatment of IBS. There were 12 studies containing a total of 1125 patients that were included in this review. Combining the data from the 12 studies showed that the TXYF was more effective than placebo in controlling IBS symptoms. The authors conclude that the Chinese herbal medicine TXYF might be effective in the treatment of IBS. Unfortunately, the quality of the 12 studies that examined this medication was very poor, and therefore a firm recommendation for the use of this Chinese herbal medicine could not be made. Finally, a larger review of the use of herbal medicines in the treatment of IBS was published in November 2005. In this review, authors gathered 75 randomized trials involving almost 8000 participants with IBS. Only three trials were considered to be of high quality, and the remaining 72 were felt to be low quality. Seventy-one different herbal medications were tested in these trials. The trials either compared the herbal remedies with placebo or were added to conventional therapies. When the herbal remedies were compared to placebo in these trials, the following herbal medicines showed a statistically significant improvement in the patient's over all symptoms: STW–5 and STW–5–II; Tibetan herbal medicine; Padma Lax; traditional Chinese formula; and Tanxie, Yaofang and Ayurdyvic preparations. No adverse reactions from herbal medications were reported in the studies. The conclusion of this large and detailed review was that some herbal medications might improve the symptoms of IBS. However, as noted, the data from many clinical trials are not of very high quality. The studies did not contain many patients, and many of them lack confirming data. It is clear that herbal medications require further examination and higher-quality clinical trials. A firm recommendation regarding their use must await those tests.

❖   **A friend of mine bought Peppermint teabags from health store and drinks a cup or two every day. He thinks it helps with his food digestion. Is that right?**

Dr. Brown: Peppermint oil has been extensively investigated in the treatment of irritable bowel syndrome. This herbal medicine is being widely used in the treatment of the symptoms of irritable bowel syndrome for its spasmolytic, carminative and sedative effects. A mixture of mints by the name of Carmint was used in a study in Iran. This mixture contained spearmint leave (Mentha spicata) and two other herb Melissa officinalis, and Coriandrun sativum and was used for improvement of symptoms of abdominal pain and bloating in subjects with irritable bowel syndrome. Patients were treated for eight weeks. This particular study showed that the frequency of abdominal pain, cramping and discomfort were significantly lower in the Carmint group than in the placebo group at the end of the treatment trial. The severity and frequency of the bloating was significantly reduced. In a recent review article in August of 2005, 16 clinical trials detailing the use of peppermint oil in the treatment of IBS were examined. Twelve of the studies were controlled by a placebo arm whereas the other four studies used a comparator of conventional therapy. Eight of the 12 placebo-controlled studies did show a statistically significant effect in favor of peppermint oil. The average overall success rate was approximately 58% for peppermint oil and only 29% for placebo. Adverse affects secondary to the use of peppermint oil were mild and short-lived but they were very specific. Patients using peppermint oil will notice heartburn and anal or peri-anal burning or discomfort. The authors concluded that peppermint oil is safe and for the most part well tolerated and appears in these studies to be effective in controlling the symptoms of irritable bowel syndrome including abdominal pain and cramping and diarrhea and/or constipation. They felt that patients in general, demonstrated improvement in the quality of life as evidenced by these clinical trials. The authors of this review may be a bit optimistic about the efficacy of peppermint oil given the quality of these studies. It should also be mentioned another review of the literature published in 1998, which only examined 8 published articles, did not show a significant role for peppermint oil in the symptom relief of IBS. In summary, peppermint oil would appear to be a safe approach and potentially effective approach to the treatment of irritable bowel syndrome complicated by abdominal pain and cramping but a firm recommendations for its use must be held back until much better clinical trials are completed.

❖ **My father-in-law uses Aloe Vera juice and encourages me to use it. He believes that this herb is great for digestive health. Is there any truth to his claim?**

Dr. Brown: Aloe Vera is a plant that can produce latex. The gel that is extracted from its leaf has been used in the treatment of a variety of gastrointestinal complaints. The majority of the work using Aloe Vera juice has been in the treatment of ulcerative colitis, where the studies vary. Recent clinical trials have suggested that Aloe Vera, when taken for four weeks, was associated with a higher clinical remission and improvement in symptoms when compared to placebo (sugar pill) in patients with ulcerative colitis. Our own studies at Rush University Medical Center with Aloe Vera juice in the setting of inflammatory bowel disease have not been as promising. There is however a single clinical trial examining the efficacy of Aloe Vera juice in the treatment of the irritable bowel syndrome. The study was published in 2006 and comes from England. Fifty-eight patients were enrolled into this clinical trial. They were treated for one month with Aloe Vera juice at a dose of the 50 milliliters taken four times a day for one month. The formulation came as pink syrup flavored with mango and the placebo given was made to match this compound in both color and flavor. The factors that were assessed in this study were abdominal pain, distention, satisfaction with their bowel habits and their overall well-being. This particular clinical trial did not show that Aloe Vera juice improves the symptoms of irritable bowel syndrome. Thirty-five percent of the patients taking the Aloe Vera juice improved whereas 22% of the patients taking placebo improved. This difference was not statistically different making this a negative study. Unfortunately, there is very little data available today to make a firm statement regarding Aloe Vera juice. The data in irritable syndrome at this time is inconclusive and does not support its use.

❖ **I saw the advertisement for live bacteria, VSL#3, in the newspaper. What is this bacterium, and will it help my IBS?**

VSL#3® is a probiotic. Probiotics are beneficial live bacteria that survive the digestion process and therefore are able to populate in the gastrointestinal tract. There are more than a million species of bacteria in our digestive tract, particularly in the large bowel. This population could be affected by diet and various disease states. It is widely believed that a proper balance of these bacteria is interconnected not only to the health of the digestive tract, but also to our sense of well-being. Several studies have shown that there are some abnormalities in the balance of the bacterial population living inside the gastrointestinal tract in some disorders including IBS. In addition, some reports claim that ingestion of live bacteria (probiotics) can restore this imbalance. There are a growing number of commercially available probiotics in the market. However, only a few of them have been standardized and tested in clinical trials. VSL#3® is one of the probiotics that contains almost a half-trillion live lactic acid bacteria that survive the journey through the GI tract and colonize the colon. The results of clinical trials on VSL#3 have provided promising effects in patients with IBS; in particular, VSL#3 reduced bloating and flatulence among these patients. As mentioned above, probiotics are live bacteria, so most of them need to be kept in the refrigerator. VSL#3® used to be available only as a powder, but recently it is being offered in pill form.

❖ **A friend of mine who has IBS told me she benefits from biofeedback. Is this a form of treatment in IBS?**

Dr. Drossman: Yes, biofeedback can be a treatment for IBS.[32] You may be referring to generalized biofeedback, which is a method where you learn to relax your body (skeletal) muscles such as the neck or back or facial muscles by observing the tension of these muscles on a computer screen. Through practice, as your muscles relax, you can achieve a general state of relaxation and this can help reduce your bowel symptoms. This is similar to other psychological treatments including hypnosis and stress management of cognitive behavioral therapy.[13, 25] Within the field of gastroenterology, there is another type of biofeedback called anorectal biofeedback. Here the probe that senses the muscle tension is applied specifically to the muscles of the pelvic floor rather than to the muscles of the body, but the goal is the same, to teach the pelvic floor muscles to relax.

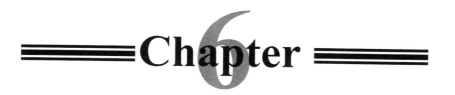

LIVING WITH IBS

<u>*In this chapter, you will learn:*</u>

✓   *What you should eat and what you should avoid.*

✓   *What the "**Dynamic Diet**" is.*

✓   *How Pregnancy affects IBS and vice versa.*

✓   *How sleep problem is related to IBS symptoms.*

✓   *How you should use the Internet to increase your understanding of IBS.*

❖ **What are dietary modifications? What should I eat? What foods should I avoid? In other words, what is the best IBS diet?**

Unfortunately, there is no good IBS diet. Consider the following example. Joe, an accountant at New life Company in Chicago, experiences abdominal pain, bloating and loose stool at the end of the fiscal year. As a result of his symptoms, he has made two visits to the emergency room. His symptoms get worse when he eats fatty and/or spicy foods. He cannot tolerate vegetables and fresh fruit. He was prescribed several medications, which temporarily relieved his symptoms. His gastroenterologist diagnosed him with IBS and recommended that he take a vacation. When he went to the Caribbean, he left all of his medication at home. Ironically, he was able to eat any type of food, without any problem. So, you be the judge. Should Joe modify his diet for the rest of his life?

❖ **So, I can eat whatever I like.**

It depends. As the previous response demonstrates, there is no diet that has been proven effective for IBS. A lot depends on the dynamic interaction between you, the food you eat, and potential environmental stressors. So, rather than proposing a fixed diet for IBS, I recommend a "Dynamic Diet."

❖ **What? A "Dynamic Diet"?!!!**

Adhering to a "Dynamic Diet" means that you determine what kind of food to include or exclude from your diet based on your current life situation as well as from your prior experiences. For example, if pickles and spices cause GI problems, you should avoid them. However, if you do not experience any difficulty with soda and fatty foods, you can include them in your diet. If your symptoms are intermittent, you should probably restrict your diet during that period of time. This is why I call it a "Dynamic Diet." You can expand your diet during symptom-free periods, but need to restrict it when you are experiencing your symptoms.

❖ **So, I suppose that pickles, spices, garlic, onions or other foods that do not bother me are harmless to my GI tract.**

Absolutely. You should know that the presence of symptoms doesn't indicate the damage to your GI tract. Indeed, these symptoms are associated with dysmotility and/or hypersensitivity, rather than mucosal damage or ulceration. These symptoms are your body's way of informing you that this particular food stimulates your GI tract and therefore should be avoided. In the absence of these warnings, there is no need to avoid those foods.

❖ **I have trouble sleeping and I feel very tired during the day. Is this related to IBS?**

Yes. There are several studies that demonstrated a close relationship between sleep and gastrointestinal symptoms. The research team at Rush University Medical Center in Chicago recently performed a study on the role of sleep in both irritable bowel syndrome and inflammatory bowel disease. The data showed that IBS subjects reported significant sleep problems in comparison with those without IBS. The findings have been accepted for publication and will be soon published in the upcoming issue of the Journal of Gastroenterology and Hepatology. Let me share an excerpt of these finding with you. IBS subjects had on average 6.0 ± 0.3 hours of sleep each night, which was less than healthy subjects (6.7 ± 0.2 hours). It took on average 50.4 ± 10 minutes for IBS subject to fall asleep, compared to the 11.6 ± 2 minutes it took healthy subjects on average to fall sleep. Overall 67% of IBS subjects reported that on one or more nights per week, it took them more than 30 minutes to fall asleep. This stands in sharp contrast to the 13% of healthy subjects who reported this problem. Sense of worry and anxiety about their disease was one of the major reasons for trouble sleeping in 29% of IBS. Eighty-eight percent of IBS subjects complained of repeated awakenings more than once or twice per night whereas only 40% of healthy subjects reported such awakenings. Repeated awakenings were most commonly attributed to abdominal pain (71%), need to use the bathroom (87%), breathing difficulty and snoring (50%), feeling too cold (61%), feeling too hot (71%) or having bad dreams (67%). Most often, subjects attributed their frequent awakenings to several of these problems. Overall, only less than 10% of IBS subjects indicated that they had slept well compared to 60% of healthy subjects. Furthermore, 54% of IBS subjects had to use a sleeping pill for sleep disturbances in the last month, while none of the healthy subjects used a sleeping pill. These data shed light on the extent of problem with sleep in IBS. Poor sleep not only is considered a source of stress, it can disturb the coping ability of patients and therefore affect the experience of symptoms including abdominal pain and fatigue. It also, could directly impact quality of life in a population that already experiences significant impairment in daily functioning, relationships and occupation. Thus, I have no doubt that poor sleep affect IBS and its symptoms. The true question is whether corrective approach toward managing sleep disturbances could change the course of IBS. I am optimistic that future research will address this question more clearly.

❖ **I observe my religious fasting days and last year when I was fasting for a few days, I noticed a significant improvement in my symptoms. Does fasting affect the symptoms of IBS?**

The studies on this subject are very limited. There is a relatively good study from Japan in which they used a 10 days fasting therapy (starvation with permission to drink water only) followed by five days of feeding and observed the symptoms after this intervention [60] . Researchers observed a significant improvement in symptoms of IBS in their study compared to control subjects with IBS who received conventional therapies. The findings of this study make sense because symptoms of the IBS is usually related to food intake or bowel movement and if you are fast for 10 days you will not have any stimuli to cause symptoms. Whether the benefits observed after a short period of fasting therapy would extend beyond the study period needs to be determined. Based on this study result you may think it is safe and helpful for your IBS to have a fasting period. However, it is hard to extrapolate the information from this study to religious fasting practice for several reasons: 1) this study showed the beneficial effect of very long fasting period and not a short one that is common in religious fasting practice that is usually 14-24 hours; and 2) in religious fasting practice, the observant usually eats a large meal (not at the typical mealtime) after fasting hours.

Thus, I would not be surprised if the fasting practice provides some relief of symptoms during fasting hours. I would also not be surprised if this relief is followed by an exacerbation of symptoms after heavy meal followed the end of the fasting hours. Overall, I think the response of each individual to the fasting period can be quiet different. Some individuals may experience more benefit from the fasting period while some may have an exaggeration of symptoms. Regardless of symptoms, there is no organic damage to the gastrointestinal tract in subjects with IBS with fasting. Based on these explanations, my suggestion is to use your own experience and see whether you are in the group that their IBS symptoms alleviate or exacerbate during this religious practice and make the call.

❖   **I am planning to get pregnant in near future. Does pregnancy affect IBS?**

As you know, IBS mainly affects young people in their reproductive years and also affects women more than men. Thus, it is not uncommon that we encounter a pregnant IBS patient in need of management in our clinic. However, there is not much information in the literature about this combination. Based on limited studies, we know almost one-third of IBS patients experience exacerbation of their constipation. Another third complains of diarrhea during their pregnancy.[61] Overall, the management of IBS during pregnancy is similar to that of non-pregnant women. There is no safe medicine during pregnancy and the IBS medications are not an exception. However, anecdotal reports of using over-the- counter medicine to relieve constipation or diarrhea did not show any harm.[62] I do not suggest using any medicine unless you really have to. There is no data in the literature that shows IBS adversely affects the course of the pregnancy or the fetus.

❖   **Do you recommend that I use the Internet to increase my understanding of IBS?**

Yes and no. There is an abundance of information regarding IBS on the Internet. However, not all of this information is accurate or useful. I recommend the following websites for further information:

http://www.aboutibs.org/. This is the website of the International Foundation of Functional Gastrointestinal Disorders (IFFGD).

http://www.talkibs.org/index.html. This is the website of the Society for Women's Health Research.

http://digestive.niddk.nih.gov/ddiseases/pubs/ibs_ez/index.htm. A service of the National Institute of Diabetes, Digestive and Kidney diseases (NIH).

http://irritablebowel.net/. This website emphasizes on psychological aspect of IBS.

http://www.mayoclinic.com/health/irritable-bowel-syndrome/DS00106. This is part of the Mayo clinic website.

http://www.emedicinehealth.com/irritable_bowel_syndrome/article_em.htm. http://en.wikipedia.org/wiki/Irritable_bowel_syndrome.

http://www.ibsassociation.org/

www.med.unc.edu/ibs

❖   **What about joining Internet or in-person support groups? Are they useful?**

Again, my answer is yes and no. On one hand, this kind of social networking can be very helpful. Participating in support groups allows you to interact with others who have the same problems as you do. It also provides you with an opportunity to hear about others' experiences and share your thoughts, concerns and questions. This may be extremely helpful and reassuring. But, on the other hand, some support groups may increase your concerns and general anxiety about IBS, due to inaccurate information or exposure to people with more severe IBS-related problems.

❖   **What is your overall advice for me?**

Now that you know more about this illness, you are already one step closer to successful management of your problem. My main goal in this book is to explain the nature of your symptoms, clarify where these symptoms are coming from, and provide you with information about what to expect when you have IBS. You also should know that you probably do not have a serious disease, like cancer, or other organic GI problem, like celiac disease or inflammatory bowel disease. Your problem is the result of dysmotility and hypersensitivity and you are capable of changing many parameters in the brain-gut axis equation. You can develop a positive attitude toward your illness and take a proactive approach toward education and treatment. Remember that, you are not the victim of this disorder, but the manager of it. You might not be able to control all of the symptoms but you can increase your coping abilities and learn how to live with some of your symptoms. You should take charge of managing your IBS and become capable of answering many of your own questions. Soon, you will be amazed how, after using these strategies the symptoms that used to annoy you may no longer bother you at all.

You should start managing your stress in any way you can. If you can't do it on your own, do not hesitate to seek help from a professional, like a psychologist. Stress and anxiety all have a negative impact on your health. So try to avoid an extremely stressful job and other life situations that cause a lot of stress. The power of saying "NO" is hard to achieve, but know your limitations and do not overwhelm yourself. When you choose to take on something, make sure it is worth it.

Add exercise to your daily routine. Even 5-10 minute of stretching before starting your day might be the key to solving many of your IBS-related problems.

Do not hesitate to use medications for your symptoms. Never fight the pain. Always consider medication as a short-term solution that provides temporary relief and gives you extra time to think of a more permanent treatment. You can also use the medicine as-needed based on disease flare-ups. Always remember that the side effects of medication might exceed their potential benefit particularly in the long run.

You can eat anything that does not bother you. Do not limit your diet based on other people's advice. Trust your GUT as the best dietitian and do not deprive yourself of your favorite food. When eating, always adhere to moderation. Add salad and fresh vegetables to your diet and supplement your diet with adequate amounts of fiber.

Search carefully to find a knowledgeable and dependable

physician and stick with him or her. Do not change physicians simply because of other people's experiences.

❖ **If I have more questions that I cannot find in this book, what should I do?**

As you noticed, this book is based on real questions that my patients have asked me during their appointments. I would be more than happy to answer your questions. I will post these questions, excluding the name of the patient, and their answers in a monthly bulletin. Thus, your question will not only help you, but also it will help others with similar concerns. I will also add selected new questions to subsequent versions of this book. Please feel free to contact me through the option of "Ask a question?" on my website: HTTP://www.IHaveIBS.com I may also send your questions to consultants who have more expertise in certain areas.

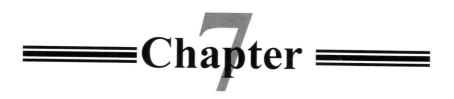

Chapter 7

IBS LATEST NEWS

<u>In this chapter, you will read the most recent news and their importance about IBS:</u>

✓ New Research in IBS

✓ New Diagnostic Tools

✓ New Treatment Options

✓ Complementary and Alternative Medicine News

✓ Living With IBS News

❖   **Enhanced Immune System in Patients with IBS**

In a study from Australia, researchers showed that the white blood cells of subjects with IBS would release more inflammatory chemicals (cytokines) at baseline and when they are stimulated with bacterial toxins. Researchers concluded that patients with diarrhea-predominant IBS have an enhanced immune system. [Gastroenterolgy, Volume 132, Issue 3, March 2007]

❖   **Is Chronic Fatigue Syndrome an Infectious Disease?**

A study from US showed for the first time that stomach biopsy might be a good method to find a dormant virus in patients with Chronic Fatigue Syndrome (CFS). This disabling condition affects a significant proportion of the work-age population and takes an expensive toll on health care costs. There is a significant correlation between this disease and IBS; however, researchers do not have a good explanation for this connection. Dr. John Chia is the co-Author of this paper and he is the father of Andrew Chia, now 24, who was diagnosed with chronic fatigue syndrome in 1997. Many researchers in the past have tried to connect the viral infections such as enterovirous to CFS, but the main way of searching for the virus was blood tests. In this study, 82% of the stomach specimens from CFS patients tested positive for enteroviral particles while only 20 percent of the samples from healthy people showed the same virus particles. It is worth mentioning that enteroviruses can cause acute respiratory and gastrointestinal infections in healthy individuals. In most cases, the enterovirus infection has a brief, self-limited course. Obtaining a stomach specimen for diagnosis of the enterovirus infection is not currently considered a standard diagnostic test. [washingtonpost.com, Thursday, September 13, 2007]

❖ **Is IBS related to intestinal bacteria?**

We live in the world full of bacteria and a world full of bacteria lives within us. Why? Because, the intestinal tract is the largest surface that connects the human body with the external environment. With more than 2000 square feet of the surface that is exposed to food and stuff that enter the body from mouth, it is not surprising that various groups of bacteria live in different parts of the GI tract. These bacteria are normal flora (good bacteria) and have a mutually helpful (symbiotic) relationship with the body. Recently, researchers have proposed that one of the culprits that cause IBS is an imbalance of good and bad bacteria in the small and large intestine. In this review, the author tried to put together a summary of the history of the research in this field and the effect of treatment with antibiotic on this condition. This field is still in its infancy and growing rather fast. [Current Treatment Opinions gastroenterology, 2007 Aug;10(4):328-37]

❖ **Can Video Capsule Endoscopy Detect Undiagnosed Cases of Crohn's Disease?**

A new report from Wake Forest University Baptist Medical Center showed capsule endoscopy detected cases of Crohn's disease of small bowel that were undiagnosed for up to 15 years. In this study, 198 cases with unexplained gastrointestinal bleeding were evaluated using video capsule endoscopy. This device takes numerous pictures from gastrointestinal lining as it travels through the digestive tract and it has been particularly useful in detecting the lesions of the small bowel where the other tests such as endoscopy or colonoscopy can not reach. In this study, Video Capsule Endoscopy diagnosed 6 cases of undiagnosed Crohn's Disease in patients who had colonoscopies and other types of tests. The most common use of this test currently includes the diagnosis of gastrointestinal bleeding with obscure source. [Healthday, November 25, 2007]

❖ **Genetic Test for Diagnosis of Lactose Intolerance**

A genetic test may replace the hydrogen breath testing for diagnosis of lactose intolerance in IBS subjects. Researchers in the Austria showed that a genetic test was 97% accurate in predicting lactose intolerance in IBS subject when it was compared with standard Hydrogen Breath Testing. Read the abstract. [Clinica Chimica Acta, Volume 383, Issues 1-2, August 2007, Pages 91-96]

❖ **Potential Stool Test for Detecting Bowel Inflammation**

A study group from Germany reported that a new diagnostic stool test that can differentiate Inflammatory Bowel Disease (IBD) from Irritable Bowel Syndrome (IBS). In this study, researchers used an assay that detected a protein (S100A12) in the fecal material that is secreted by white blood cells and the level is increased in stool of IBD subjects. (Prior studies used another protein (calprotectin) in the stool for the same reason with some success). The accuracy of this test in differentiating IBS from IBD is relatively high (sensitivity of

86% and specificity of 96%) and could be an excellent noninvasive tool in diagnosis of gastrointestinal disorders. [GUT, 2007 Dec;56(12):1706-13]

❖   **New Option for the Treatment of IBS with Constipation is on the Horizon**

Dynogen Pharmaceuticals, Inc. announced the start of an early phase of clinical research of their new medicine, which promotes the motility of the gastrointestinal tract. The name of this new medicine is DDP733 (pumosetrag). In this new trial, the medicine is used in a randomized, double blind, placebo-controlled fashion. This means that neither patients nor doctors who are involved in patient care are aware whether the patient is taking the active medicine or the placebo. This medicine can be a potential agent that can fill the vacuum generated in the market for the treatment of IBS with constipation after withdrawal of Zelnorm from the market due to safety issues. [Medical News Today, 09 Nov 2007]

❖   **Is IBS an Infectious Disease?**

A new study released by Associated Press showed that an antibiotic called Rifaximin could improve the symptoms of IBS. This study is another piece of evidence in a new campaign on the role of bacteria in IBS. There are tons of bacteria in our gastrointestinal tract, which are predominantly located in large intestine. It is believed that an imbalance in the type of bacteria or overgrowth of bacteria in the small bowel, which is usually a germ free environment, could contribute to symptoms of IBS. [forbes.com 27 Sep 2007]

❖   **A New Medicine on Horizon for Patients with IBS**

Sucampo Pharmaceuticals submitted a supplemental new drug application to the FDA to market their drug, Amitiza®, currently used for chronic constipation, to patients with IBS with constipation. Clinical trials have shown that patients receiving lubiprostone were twice as likely to achieve an overall response. [Medical News Today 13 Jul 2007]

❖   **Is Zelnorm® on Its Way Back to Market?**

Novartis, the pharmaceutical company that produces Zelnorm®, is now allowed to distribute the drug on a limited basis for treatment of IBS. Last spring, Zelnorm® was taken off the market after a few cardiovascular events (stroke and heart attack) in patients taking the drug. The withdrawal of Zelnorm® limited the treatment options of patients with constipation dominant IBS. The current use of the medicine is restricted to only a limited group of patients, women under the age of 55, which fit the criteria set by the FDA. [Medical News Today 28 Jul 2007]

❖   **Natural Clay in Treatment of Diarrhea in IBS**

A group of researchers in Taiwan showed that natural clay named Dioctahedral Smectite (DS) was useful in treating diarrhea-predominant irritable bowel syndrome. The effect was proved to be superior to placebo in an eight-week trial. [J. Gastroenterology and Hepatology, Volume 22 Issue 12, page 2266-2272]

❖   **Treatment of IBS with Osteopathy**

Osteopathy is a manual treatment to relieve body complaints, which relies on mobilizing and manipulating body. In a recent study in the Netherlands, a group of researchers showed that osteopathic treatment helped patients with IBS with their symptoms. In this study, 68% of patients in the osteopathy group noted definite overall improvement in symptoms and 27% showed slight improvement. In the control group who did not receive osteopathic treatment, only 18% noted definite improvement, 59% showed slight improvement, and in 17% experienced worsening of symptoms. A significant increase in the quality of life score was only observed in the osteopathic treatment group. The authors concluded that osteopathic therapy is a promising alternative in the treatment of patients with IBS. [J. Gastroenterology and Hepatology, 2007 Sep;22(9):1394-8]

❖   **IBS Patients Are at Higher Risk for Unrelated Common Disorders**

IBS patients appear to show a general amplification of disease incidence. The disorders that are the most common in the general population are similarly common in IBS patients with higher relative incidence. These disorders do not share their origin with IBS and include diseases such as upper respiratory tract infection, ear infection, stroke and many other common disorders. The reason for higher incidence for these disorders in IBS is not known. The authors concluded this might be due to more symptoms reporting and consultation rather than shared etiology of the disorders. [American Journal of Gastroenterology, Volume 102 Issue 12 Page 2767-2776,

December 2007]

❖   **Skin Allergy Testing and IBS**

Prior investigators have shown that individual foods can trigger symptoms in some patients 15-67% of IBS subjects may benefit from dietary manipulation. In this study, researchers used skin allergy testing and showed that 25% of 100 cases with IBS had positive skin allergy test to specific food. This was much higher than similar allergy in general population (1 in 100 cases). This study did not test to see if elimination of the specific diet would result in improvement of symptoms. [J Clinical Gastroenterology, 2007;102:1-6]

❖   **Stress and Gut Bacteria**

In a recent commentary paper that was published in GUT journal, the details of the changes in bacteria behavior with human stress hormones were explained. There are several pieces of evidence that bacteria change their virulence (attacking properties) when they sense human stress hormones such as Norepinephrin. This may open a new avenue in the investigation of the role of stress on GI tract and explain why the population of bacteria may differ in those patients with IBS. [GUT, 2007 Aug;56(8):1037-8]

❖   **How do the bacteria in my gut affect my IBS?**

A new study from Finland showed that the fecal bacteria of patients with IBS differ significantly from that of healthy subjects. In this study, the researcher used a very accurate technique to detect the strains of bacteria. This technique is far more advanced than culture technique, which has been used in the past for detection and identification of intestinal bacteria. The relevance of this new finding to the symptoms and treatment of IBS is still unknown. [Gastroenterology, 2007 Jul;133(1):24-33]

❖ **Aged Cheese can be better tolerated by individuals with lactose intolerance**

Good news for cheese lovers who can not have their favorite food! Lactose intolerance is caused by a lack of the lactase enzyme in their small bowel. Based on this study, aged cheese contains less lactose, as the bacteria has had more time to work on its lactose. For example, hard, aged cheeses such as cheddar, parmesan or gruyere has less lactose than more fresh cheeses such as Port Salut or mozzarella. This is because most of the lactose found in CHEESE winds up in the whey, rather than curd, and the lactose left in the curd is digested by the same bacteria that transforms the new curds into cheese. [Sun-Sentinel.com, Nov 26, 2007]

❖ **Bacteria with benefits**

When most people think of bacteria, they think of sickness. However, products containing bacteria are a growing trend in the health food industry. These products contain "healthy" bacteria, called probiotics, which are similar to those already present in the digestive tract. The probiotics are intended to improve the function of the digestive system, and a number of people claim the products make a difference. While the benefit of probiotics has not been scientifically determined, there are over 150 probiotic products currently available to the U.S.

market. [Washington Post, Dec. 10, 2007]

❖ **"BUGS" Are They Friends or Foe?**

For years, we've been killing bacteria with any measure we could, using all kinds of antibacterial agents such as antibiotics, germicide wipes, antiseptics, bleach, germicide tissue papers, food processing and refrigeration. However, new data is emerging that shows that bacteria could be our friends. In this brief article, the writer explores the role of good bacteria in our life and questions several experts in this field. "We all have unique bacteria profiles, like fingerprints, with our own ratio of good-to-bad bacteria" the article says. In this article, the collective experts believe that we should be more friendly toward good bacteria and try to preserve them. This may be through the use of probiotics (good bacteria in our diet) or other means. [Asbury Park Press Nov. 11, 2007]

❖ **IBS is a significant cause of lost work hours**

Researchers from Mayo Clinic College of Medicine presented their research data at the recent American College of Gastroenterology annual meeting in Philadelphia. The research showed that patients with functional gastrointestinal disorders, and in particular, patients with constipation predominant IBS, lose 10.3 hours of their work time during each work week (40 hours). Considering the large population with IBS, it is not surprising how this problem translates into a large financial loss to the workforce all around the world. [Forbes Oct 16, 2007]

❖   **Food Intolerance vs. Food Allergy**

Many people have sensitivities to certain kinds of foods, which can cause a range of symptoms. But, what is a food allergy and what is food intolerance? The difference is in the body's response to the food. Allergies are the more severe of the two: the food triggers the immune system, releasing immunoglobulin E antibodies. The resulting symptoms, including hives and respiratory difficulties, appear quickly. Food intolerance, however, is the more common of the two and does not involve the immune system. Symptoms include diarrhea and bloating. A doctor can help determine the cause of food sensitivities. [Nutrition Horizon, Dec. 10, 2007]

❖   **SIBO or IBS? The answer is a breath away**

Shortly after birth, the human digestive tract is populated by many kinds of bacteria. In some cases, the bacteria become overly abundant, resulting in small intestinal bacterial overgrowth (SIBO). The symptoms of SIBO are similar to those of IBS, and a new test can easily determine the cause of the discomfort. The so-called "Breath Test" detects abnormal amounts of hydrogen in exhaled air, which may indicate the presence of SIBO. The overgrowth can then be treated with antibiotics. [Medical News Today, Dec. 20, 2007]

❖   **Can I Eventually Outgrow IBS?**

Maybe. The researchers from Mayo Clinic reported data on 1,365 IBS patients that were followed for an average of 12 years. They found that the shape of symptoms changes from one form of functional bowel disorder to another form, but only in a minority of the cases do the symptoms disappear completely. In this study, over a 12 year period, 20% of subjects had the similar symptoms over the follow-up period, 40% did not have their initial symptoms but developed newer symptoms, and 40% completely recovered from their IBS symptoms. [Gastroenterology, 2007 Sep;133(3):799-807]

I hope this educational material has helped you to learn more about Irritable Bowel Syndrome. Your knowledge about the exact nature of this problem is the most important step in taking your active role in the management of this problem.

If you want to be a competent manager of your IBS, you should keep up with new information constantly and reinforce the information you have already obtained. You must make education a continuous habit.

Congratulations in completing this educational material and being one step closer to a successful IBS management. I wish you the best of luck.

Dr. Farhadi

LITERATURE CITATIONS

1. Drossman, D.A., et al., U.S. householder survey of functional gastrointestinal disorders. Prevalence, sociodemography, and health impact. Dig Dis Sci, 1993. *38(9): p. 1569-80.*

2. Farhadi, A., et al., Irritable bowel syndrome: an update on therapeutic modalities. Expert Opin Investig Drugs, 2001. *10(7): p. 1211-22.*

3. Thompson, W.G., et al., Irritable bowel syndrome in general practice: prevalence, characteristics, and referral. Gut, 2000. *46(1): p. 78-82.*

4. Thompson, W.G. and K.W. Heaton, Functional bowel disorders in apparently healthy people. Gastroenterology, 1980. *79(2): p. 283-8.*

5. Talley, N.J., Irritable bowel syndrome: definition, diagnosis and epidemiology. Baillieres Best Pract Res Clin Gastroenterol, 1999. *13(3): p. 371-84.*

6. Saito, Y.A., et al., A comparison of the Rome and Manning criteria for case identification in epidemiological investigations of irritable bowel syndrome. Am J Gastroenterol, 2000. *95(10): p. 2816-24.*

7. Talley, N.J., et al., Medical costs in community subjects with irritable bowel syndrome. Gastroenterology, 1995. *109(6): p. 1736-41.*

8. Talley, N.J., A.L. Weaver, and A.R. Zinsmeister, Impact of functional dyspepsia on quality of life. Dig Dis Sci, 1995. *40(3): p. 584-9.*

9. Jones, R. and S. Lydeard, Irritable bowel syndrome in the general population. Bmj, 1992. *304(6819): p. 87-90.*

10. Manning, A.P., et al., Towards positive diagnosis of the irritable bowel. Br Med J, 1978. *2(6138): p. 653-4.*

11. Drossman, D.A., The Rome criteria process: diagnosis and legitimization of irritable bowel syndrome. Am J Gastroenterol, 1999. *94(10): p. 2803-7.*

12. Longstreth GF, T.W., Chey WD, Houghton LA, Mearin F, Spiller RC., Functional Bowel Disorders. 3rd Edition ed. Rome III: The Functional Gastrointestinal Disorders, ed. C.E. Drossman DA, Delvaux M, Spiller RC, Talley NJ, Thompson WG et al. 2006: McLean, VA: Degnon Associates, Inc.

13. Drossman DA, C.E., Delvaux M, Spiller RC, Talley NJ, Thompson WG et al., Rome III: The Functional Gastrointestinal Disorders. 3rd Edition ed ed. 2006, McLean, VA: Degnon Associates, Inc.

14. Longstreth, G.F., et al., Functional bowel disorders. Gastroenterology, 2006. *130(5): p. 1480-91.*

15. Su, Y.C., et al., The association between Helicobacter pylori infection and functional dyspepsia in patients with irritable bowel syndrome. Am J Gastroenterol, 2000. *95(8): p. 1900-5.*

16. O'Mahony, L., et al., Lactobacillus and bifidobacterium in irritable bowel syndrome: symptom responses and relationship to cytokine profiles. Gastroenterology, 2005. *128(3): p. 541-51.*

17. Santos, J., et al., Role of mast cells in chronic stress induced colonic epithelial barrier dysfunction in the rat. Gut, 2001. *48(5): p. 630-6.*

18. Santos, J., et al., Chronic stress impairs rat growth and jejunal epithelial barrier function: role of mast cells. Am J Physiol Gastrointest Liver Physiol, 2000. *278(6): p. G847-54.*

19. Farhadi, A.F., JZ. Keshavarzian, A., Mucosal mast cells are pivotal elements in inflammatory bowel disease that connect the dots: Stress, intestinal hyperpermeability and inflammation. World Journal of Gastroenterology, 2007.

20. Farhadi, A., et al., Heightened responses to stressors in patients with inflammatory bowel disease. Am J Gastroenterol, 2005. *100(8): p. 1796-804.*

21. Barbara, G., et al., Mast cell-dependent excitation of visceral-nociceptive sensory neurons in irritable bowel syndrome. Gastroenterology, 2007. *132(1): p. 26-37.*

22. Barbara, G., et al., Activated mast cells in proximity to colonic nerves correlate with abdominal pain in irritable bowel syndrome. Gastroenterology, 2004. *126(3): p. 693-702.*

23.   *Jakate, S., et al., Mastocytic enterocolitis: increased mucosal mast cells in chronic intractable diarrhea. Arch Pathol Lab Med, 2006. **130**(3): p. 362-7.*

24.   *Creed F, L.R., Bradley L, Fransisconi C, Drossman DA, Naliboff B et al., Psychosocial Aspects of Functional Gastrointestinal Disorders. 3rd Edition ed ed. Rome III: The Functional Gastrointestinal Disorders, ed. C.E. Drossman DA, Delvaux M, Spiller RC, Talley NJ, Thompson WG et al. 2006, McLean, VA: Degnon Associates, Inc.*

25.   *Levy, R.L., et al., Psychosocial aspects of the functional gastrointestinal disorders. Gastroenterology, 2006. **130**(5): p. 1447-58.*

26.   *Drossman, D.A., et al., Health status by gastrointestinal diagnosis and abuse history. Gastroenterology, 1996. **110**(4): p. 999-1007.*

27.   *Leserman, J. and D.A. Drossman, Relationship of abuse history to functional gastrointestinal disorders and symptoms: some possible mediating mechanisms. Trauma Violence Abuse, 2007. **8**(3): p. 331-43.*

28.   *Tobin MC, M.B., Farhadi A, Demeo MT, Bansal PJ, Keshavarzian A, Atopic irritable Bowel syndrome: A novel subgroup of irritable bowel syndrome with allergic manifestation. Annals of Allergy, Asthma and Immunology, 2008. **100**: p. 49-53.*

29.   *Liebregts, T., et al., Immune activation in patients with irritable bowel syndrome. Gastroenterology, 2007. **132**(3): p. 913-20.*

30.   *O'Donnell LJ, V.J., Heaton KW, Detection of pseudodiarrhoea by simple clinical assessment of intestinal transit rate. BMJ, 1990. **17;300**(6722):439-40.*

31.   *Bharucha, A.E., et al., Functional anorectal disorders. Gastroenterology, 2006. **130**(5): p. 1510-8.*

32.   *Chiarioni, G., et al., Biofeedback is superior to laxatives for normal transit constipation due to pelvic floor dyssynergia. Gastroenterology, 2006. **130**(3): p. 657-64.*

33.   *Salvioli, B., et al., Impaired small bowel gas propulsion in patients with bloating during intestinal lipid infusion. Am J Gastroenterol, 2006. **101**(8): p. 1853-7.*

34.   *Pimentel, M., E.J. Chow, and H.C. Lin, Eradication of small intestinal bacterial overgrowth reduces symptoms of irritable bowel syndrome. Am J Gastroenterol, 2000. **95**(12): p. 3503-6.*

35.   *Posserud, I., et al., Small intestinal bacterial overgrowth in patients with irritable bowel syndrome. Gut, 2007. **56**(6): p. 802-8.*

36.   *Walters, B. and S.J. Vanner, Detection of bacterial overgrowth in IBS using the lactulose H2 breath test: comparison with 14C-D-xylose and healthy controls. Am J Gastroenterol, 2005. **100**(7): p. 1566-70.*

37.   *Blanchard, E.B., et al., Relaxation training as a treatment for irritable bowel syndrome. Biofeedback Self Regul, 1993. **18**(3): p. 125-32.*

38.   *Shaw, G., et al., Stress management for irritable bowel syndrome: a controlled trial. Digestion, 1991. **50**(1): p. 36-42.*

39.   *Barak, N., R. Ishai, and E. Lev-Ran, [Biofeedback treatment of irritable bowel syndrome]. Harefuah, 1999. **137**(3-4): p. 105-7, 175.*

40.   *Leahy, A., et al., Computerised biofeedback games: a new method for teaching stress management and its use in irritable bowel syndrome. J R Coll Physicians Lond, 1998. **32**(6): p. 552-6.*

41.   *Guthrie, E., et al., A controlled trial of psychological treatment for the irritable bowel syndrome. Gastroenterology, 1991. **100**(2): p. 450-7.*

42.   *Blanchard, E.B., et al., Two controlled evaluations of multicomponent psychological treatment of irritable bowel syndrome. Behav Res Ther, 1992. **30**(2): p. 175-89.*

43.   *Houghton, L.A., D.J. Heyman, and P.J. Whorwell, Symptomatology, quality of life and economic features of irritable bowel syndrome--the effect of hypnotherapy. Aliment Pharmacol Ther, 1996. **10**(1): p. 91-5.*

44.   *Whorwell, P.J., A. Prior, and E.B. Faragher, Controlled trial of hypnotherapy in the treatment of severe refractory irritable-bowel syndrome. Lancet, 1984. **2**(8414): p. 1232-4.*

45.   *Read, N.W., Harnessing the patient's powers of recovery: the role of the psychotherapies in the irritable bowel syndrome. Baillieres Best Pract Res Clin Gastroenterol, 1999. **13**(3): p. 473-87.*

46. Milo, R., *Use of the peripheral dopamine antagonist, domperidone, in the management of gastro-intestinal symptoms in patients with irritable bowel syndrome.* Curr Med Res Opin, 1980. **6**(9): p. 577-84.

47. Van Outryve, M., et al., *"Prokinetic" treatment of constipation-predominant irritable bowel syndrome: a placebo-controlled study of cisapride.* J Clin Gastroenterol, 1991. **13**(1): p. 49-57.

48. Cann, P.A., et al., *Role of loperamide and placebo in management of irritable bowel syndrome (IBS).* Dig Dis Sci, 1984. **29**(3): p. 239-47.

49. Camilleri, M., *Management of the irritable bowel syndrome.* Gastroenterology, 2001. **120**(3): p. 652-68.

50. Camilleri, M., *Pharmacology and clinical experience with alosetron.* Expert Opin Investig Drugs, 2000. **9**(1): p. 147-59.

51. Poynard, T., C. Regimbeau, and Y. Benhamou, *Meta-analysis of smooth muscle relaxants in the treatment of irritable bowel syndrome.* Aliment Pharmacol Ther, 2001. **15**(3): p. 355-61.

52. Muller-Lissner, S.A., et al., *Tegaserod, a 5-HT(4) receptor partial agonist, relieves symptoms in irritable bowel syndrome patients with abdominal pain, bloating and constipation.* Aliment Pharmacol Ther, 2001. **15**(10): p. 1655-66.

53. Coremans, G., et al., *Prucalopride is effective in patients with severe chronic constipation in whom laxatives fail to provide adequate relief. Results of a double-blind, placebo-controlled clinical trial.* Digestion, 2003. **67**(1-2): p. 82-9.

54. Malcolm, A., et al., *Towards identifying optimal doses for alpha-2 adrenergic modulation of colonic and rectal motor and sensory function.* Aliment Pharmacol Ther, 2000. **14**(6): p. 783-93.

55. Hasler, W.L., H.C. Soudah, and C. Owyang, *Somatostatin analog inhibits afferent response to rectal distention in diarrhea-predominant irritable bowel patients.* J Pharmacol Exp Ther, 1994. **268**(3): p. 1206-11.

56. Julia, V., O. Morteau, and L. Bueno, *Involvement of neurokinin 1 and 2 receptors in viscerosensitive response to rectal distension in rats.* Gastroenterology, 1994. **107**(1): p. 94-102.

57. Laird, J.M., et al., *Responses of rat spinal neurons to distension of inflamed colon: role of tachykinin NK2 receptors.* Neuropharmacology, 2001. **40**(5): p. 696-701.

58. Mannion, R.J., et al., *Neurotrophins: peripherally and centrally acting modulators of tactile stimulus-induced inflammatory pain hypersensitivity.* Proc Natl Acad Sci U S A, 1999. **96**(16): p. 9385-90.

59. Crowell, M.D., et al., *Antidepressants in the treatment of irritable bowel syndrome and visceral pain syndromes.* Curr Opin Investig Drugs, 2004. **5**(7): p. 736-42.

60. Kanazawa, M. and S. Fukudo, *Effects of fasting therapy on irritable bowel syndrome.* Int J Behav Med, 2006. **13**(3): p. 214-20.

61. Hasler, W.L., *The irritable bowel syndrome during pregnancy.* Gastroenterol Clin North Am, 2003. **32**(1): p. 385-406, viii.

62. Bruno, M., *Irritable bowel syndrome and inflammatory bowel disease in pregnancy.* J Perinat Neonatal Nurs, 2004. **18**(4): p. 341-50; quiz 351-2.

Made in the USA
Lexington, KY
18 September 2010